MW01101821

The Blue Line Incision and Refractive Phacoemulsification

The Blue Line Incision and Refractive Phacoemulsification

Kurt A. Buzard, MD, FACS
Buzard Eye Institute
Las Vegas, Nevada

Miles H. Friedlander, MD, FACS
Tulane University
New Orleans, Louisiana

Jean-Luc Febbraro, MD
Rothschild Foundation
Paris, France

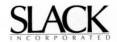

SLACK
INCORPORATED

an innovative information, education and management company
6900 Grove Road • Thorofare, NJ 08086

Publisher: John H. Bond
Editorial Director: Amy E. Drummond
Senior Associate Editor: Jennifer Stewart
Illustrations on cover, chapters 2, 5, 6, 10 by: Stephen Gordon

The procedures and practices described in this book should be implemented in a manner consistent with the professional standards set for the circumstances that apply in each specific situation. Every effort has been made to confirm the accuracy of the information presented and to correctly relate gen-erally accepted practices. The author, editor, and publisher cannot accept responsibility for errors or exclusions or for the outcome of the application of the material presented herein. There is no expressed or implied warranty of this book or information imparted by it.

Care has been taken to ensure that drug selection and dosages are in accordance with currently accepted/recommended practice. Due to continuing research, changes in government policy and reg-ulations, and various effects of drug reactions and interactions, it is recommended that the reader review all materials and literature provided for each drug, especially those that are new or not fre-quently used.

Any review or mention of specific companies or products is not intended as an endorsement by the author or the publisher.

The Blue Line Incision and Refractive Phacoemulsification / [edited by] Kurt Buzard.
    p. ; cm.
    Includes bibliographical references and index.
    ISBN 1-55642-481-7 (alk. paper)
    1. Cataract--Surgery. 2. Phacoemulsification. I. Buzard, Kurt. II. Friedlander, Miles.
    III. Febbraro, Jean Luc.
    [DNLM: 1. Cataract Extraction. 2. Phacoemulsification--methods. WW 260 B658 2000]
    RE451 .B58 2000
    617.7'42059--dc21
                                                           00-056306

Printed in Canada.

Published by: SLACK Incorporated
                  6900 Grove Road
                  Thorofare, NJ 08086 USA
                  Telephone: 856-848-1000
                  Fax: 856-853-5991
                  www.slackbooks.com

Last digit is print number: 10 9 8 7 6 5 4 3 2 1

Dedication

It is with profound humility that the authors dedicate this text to José Ignacio Barraquer. For those of us who were privileged to know Dr. Barraquer and to have been invited to study at his side, he will always be the teacher whose example we sought to emulate, the friend whose advice we treasured, and the giant among his peers who shared his gifts so freely. All whose lives he touched are richer for having known him.

Miles H. Friedlander, MD, FACS
Kurt A. Buzard, MD, FACS

I dedicate this book to my mentors, Daniéle Aron-Rosa and Jean-Jacques Aron in France, and to Kurt Buzard and Miles Friedlander in the United States.

It has been an honor and privilege to study at their sides during my residency and fellowship. Each has in his own way made an invaluable contribution to both my professional and private lives. I remain in awe of their clinical and surgical expertise, their contagious passion for ophthalmology, and their unwavering commitment to the pursuit of excellence.

You have allowed me to spend all these precious years with you, during which, you have given me far more than I have given you. But please be patient, this is a work in progress.

Jean-Luc Febbraro, MD

Contents

About the Authors

Kurt A. Buzard, MD, FACS

Dr. Kurt Buzard earned his MD from Northwestern University and holds an advanced degree in physics from Stanford University. Dr. Buzard's background includes a 4-year residency at Jules Stein Institute and UCLA followed by a fellowship in corneal and refractive surgery at Manhattan Eye, Ear, Nose and Throat Hospital, where he studied corneal disorders and refractive surgery under the tutelage of Dr. Richard Troutman. He further studied under the supervision of José Barraquer, MD, in Bogota, Colombia.

Dr. Buzard has conducted extensive research into corneal and refractive disorders, has written extensively on these subjects, and contributed to the scientific advancement of treatment for these disorders.

Dr. Buzard has been in practice in Las Vegas since 1986. His practice is limited to corneal/refractive and cataract surgery. He is a clinical assistant professor of ophthalmology at the University of Nevada School of Medicine and Tulane University School of Medicine in New Orleans.

Miles H. Friedlander, MD, FACS

Dr. Friedlander became actively involved in refractive surgery under the tutelage of Dr. José Barraquer. After attending Dr. Barraquer's second instructional course in keratophakia and keratomileusis in Bogota, Colombia in September 1977, he returned to New Orleans, where he performed his first case of keratophakia 2 months later. In 1978, José Barraquer, Richard Troutman, and he founded the International Society of Refractive Keratoplasty to provide a worldwide forum for the scientific investigation and advancement of refractive surgery. He has organized and participated in national and international instructional courses and seminars ranging from the classic Barraquer procedures and their subsequent laser adaptations, as well as radial and astigmatic keratotomies, and most recently, phakic refractive surgery. He has contributed chapters to eight refractive surgery books and has authored over 40 articles in ophthalmic refractive journals. He has served on the editorial board of the *Journal of Cataract and Refractive Surgery* and is currently on the editorial board of the *Journal of Refractive Surgery*.

Dr. Friedlander graduated from Louisiana State Medical School and completed his ophthalmology residency at Tulane University in New Orleans. He is professor of ophthalmology at Tulane University Medical Center and is a consultant to Eye Care Associates. He performs refractive surgery at the Eye Care Institute in Metairie, La.

Jean-Luc Febbraro, MD

Dr. Febbraro completed a 1-year fellowship in corneal and refractive surgery at the Buzard Institute in 1999, sponsored by Tulane University, New Orleans, La. During this period, he had the opportunity to advance his knowledge of anterior segment surgery, increase his research experience under the tutelage of Drs. Buzard and Friedlander, and contribute to the publication of several papers in refractive surgery.

Dr. Febbraro obtained his doctorate of medicine at Turin University, Turin, Italy, began his residency at Milan University, Milan, Italy, and completed his residency at the Ambrose Pare Hospital and Rothschild Foundation in Paris. His fellowship in corneal and refractive surgery was accomplished at Paris VII University. During this 3-year fellowship training, he participated with Dr. Daniéle Aron-Rosa in numerous prospective clinical trials for European and US Food and Drug Administration evaluation, as well as in the development of excimer laser surgery, including photorefractive keratectomy, laser in situ keratomileusis, and refractive lensectomy.

Contributing Authors

Brannon Aden, MD
New Orleans, Louisiana

Daniéle Aron-Rosa, MD
Paris, France

Kurt A. Buzard, MD, FACS
Las Vegas, Nevada

Paul Ernest, MD
Jackson, Michigan

Jean-Luc Febbraro, MD
Paris, France

Miles H. Friedlander, MD, FACS
New Orleans, Louisiana

Nicole S. Granet, BA
New Orleans, Louisiana

Maurice E. John, MD
Jeffersonville, Indiana

Randall Noblitt, OD
Jeffersonville, Indiana

Lee H. Novick, MD
Newport Coast, California

Luis E. Remus, PhD, MD
New Orleans, Louisiana

Richard C. Troutman, MD, FACS, FRCOphth
New York, New York

R. Bruce Wallace, III, MD, FACS
Alexandria, Louisiana

Preface

It has been a pleasure writing this book with my coauthors Miles Friedlander, MD and Jean-Luc Febbraro, MD. I have a long-standing personal relationship with Miles that spans the past 15 years. He was among those who had the initial confidence to support me in my early career. Likewise, it was a pleasure to work with Jean-Luc Febbraro, who I anticipate will make significant contributions to ophthalmology, as his mentors would expect. I wish to acknowledge Richard Troutman, MD, who continues to be a mentor and has unfailingly supported me in my career over the years.

I wish to acknowledge the participation of our contributors: Brannon Aden, Paul Ernest, Maurice John, Daniéle Aron-Rosa, Richard Troutman, and Bruce Wallace. These contributing authors have each distinguished themselves in their respective fields and have made significant contributions to ophthalmology over the years. We consider ourselves fortunate that they agreed to contribute to this book.

I would like to acknowledge and thank Brett Bertram, who has spent months editing, organizing, and integrating the material presented in this book. His expertise with the English language has made the material presented in this book more readable and concise than the form in which it was presented to him.

I wish to thank Nicole Granet Friedlander for continued support and friendship over the years, and my wife, Carol, who continues to spend many hours encouraging and organizing these projects. We hope our efforts will encourage you to use these techniques and ideas in your ophthalmology practice.

I would also like to thank SLACK editors Viktoria Kristiansson, Lauren Plummer, Jennifer Stewart, and Debra Toulson for their patience and diligence, and finally, my appreciation to SLACK Incorporated for the opportunity to present this material in print.

Kurt Buzard, MD, FACS

1 Introduction

Kurt A. Buzard, MD, FACS

During the past 20 years, there has been a remarkable flurry of activity revolving around the creation of the cataract incision and cataract surgery in general. By fortune and coincidence, I have had the privilege to live through this time and know first-hand many of the architects of this revolution, as have many of you who read this book. When I began my residency at UCLA in 1980, intracapsular 11-mm incisions were still commonplace and part of the curriculum. The faculty, with a few notable exceptions, still practiced extracapsular cataract surgery with a 9-mm incision, most often without an intraocular lens (IOL); and phacoemulsification was performed with the original cavitron unit, when "tuning" the machine really meant holding it up to your ear and listening to the pitch produced by adjusting the machine. Since that time, the changes have been so frequent and continuous that it is sometimes difficult to fathom the implications of the accumulation of these changes. This book is an attempt to look at lens-based surgery in a new refractive light: in a sense, to make a statement that refractive cataract surgery can now be a reality with the right techniques and attitude.

With reductions in incision size, the introduction of phacoemulsification, and further reductions in size allowed by the use of foldable intraocular lenses, the cataract incision has gradually become smaller and smaller, reaching what might have once seemed unbelievable: the sub 2-mm incision. At this point the basic architecture of the incision has become an issue of discussion. Prior to this time the scleral tunnel incision had been the primary means of creating the entry into the eye, usually beginning 2 to 3 mm behind the limbus and proceeding in a step fashion into the clear cornea and then into the anterior chamber. While this incision was quite satisfactory in terms of stability and bursting pressure, efficiency was limited primarily due to the metal knives usually used to create the incision and the perceived need for a peritomy to avoid chemosis. This could require extended time and necessitate a peritomy with subsequent cautery with the potential of induced astigmatism from the cautery. Even at this time, however, the benefits of a scleral tunnel incision extending into the cornea were apparent and taught. The surgery was facilitated by less iris prolapse and fewer problems with pressure, even though the underlying theory of a self-sealing incision was still many years away.

Primarily as a result of the desire for increased efficiency, the external cataract incision began to migrate into the clear cornea. Several advantages to this incision construction technique became apparent. First, even with metal knives, the incision could be created relatively quickly, thus increasing the efficiency of incision creation. Second, by creating an anterior incision entering the anterior chamber well within the clear cornea, technical improvements in the cataract surgery became apparent and a theory was proposed to explain these advantages. The problem of iris prolapse became less common. Control of the anterior chamber was improved with modifications to the phacoemulsification tip, thus improving control of the angle of approach during phacoemulsification and giving certain advantages to the removal of the nucleus.

As a result of the shift to the clear cornea approach, several problems also became apparent. First, if the tunnel length in the cornea was too long, stria would develop, obscuring detail during cataract removal and making the surgery more difficult. Second, since the clear cornea incision had a very fragile anterior lip (consisting of corneal tissue) and could not be grasped with the forceps, stabilization of the globe became more complicated, requiring either a ring, insertion of instruments in the second opening, or a forceps grasping the conjunctiva. Therefore, some of the efficiency gains in the creation of the incision were compromised in stabilizing the globe. The incision needed to be performed in a temporal location since the longer incision tended to be closer to the optical axis superiorly. This temporal location was not mechanically advantageous in terms of ocular integrity and the possibility of "fish-mouthing" with relatively small construction errors led to periodic wound incompetence. In addition, the clear corneal incision has a tendency to create both regular and irregular astigmatism, an advantage for patients with against-the-rule astigmatism but still less than optimal for true control of the refractive aspects of lens-based surgeries. Discussion of the need to abandon the "groove" to begin the incision and the question of its contribution to induced astigmatism only made construction more difficult, since the anterior corneal lip became even more fragile and prone to leakage. Finally, the positioning of the incision entirely within the cornea made this relatively fragile tissue the recipient of the majority of energy transferred from the tip to surrounding tissue, resulting in endothelial loss and even corneal "burn" if the case was extended.

It is in this context that Paul Ernest and Thomas Neuhann began to re-examine the clear corneal incision. Ernest was particularly concerned about the slow healing of the corneal incision and the mechanics of a strong incision. His work showed the importance of a relatively square incision and the wound healing benefits of entering through the "bloody limbus." The implication was that moving more posteriorly had significant benefits in terms of safety and that some compromise needed to be made between the efficiency of clear cornea and the safety and flexibility of the scleral tunnel incision. In addition, for refractive purposes, the astigmatic stability offered by a scleral incision with the "funnel" described by Koch offered more flexibility and predictability than the clear corneal incision with its induction of regular and irregular astigmatism. Additionally, since most of the trauma of ultrasound and manipulation were borne by the relatively robust scleral tissue, 1 day postoperative vision was improved, leading to greater satisfaction in terms of refractive result.

We present this book, which describes the transconjunctival "blue line" incision, in context with "refractive phacoemulsification." The elements have been in place for some time—Ernest and Neuhann provide the context—and surgeons around the world have used similar incisions. What remains is the need to make the benefits clear and to encourage transition to this excellent technique. The emergence of long cataract diamonds with truncated tips from Mastel (Rapid City, SD) have made the incision technically accessible to almost everyone. With its short learning curve, the transition itself should be nearly painless for surgeons practicing clear corneal and scleral tunnel surgery alike. In addition, we bring together a small compendium of ideas, techniques, and instruments that we believe form the basis of a revolution in the expectations of both surgeon and patient with respect to refractive outcomes in lens-based surgery. Taken alone each technique is of interest; taken as a group, we believe that with the tools and techniques readily available, truly refractive lens surgery can now be a reality. It is only necessary to look at cataract and lens exchange surgery in a new light rather than ignore 1 diopter of astigmatism or a small spherical error, to attack these problems directly, and delight both patient and surgeon with cumulative results of 20/40 or better without correction. Small refractive errors need not be ignored and techniques presented in this book show how relatively simple changes and procedures can lead to freedom from spectacle correction in the vast majority of lens-based surgeries.

Stop for a moment and consider the time spent with patients prescribing temporary glasses after surgery and the concern patients may have in proceeding to the second eye with significant anisotropia and/or other refractive problems. Imagine patients integrated into a practice of laser-assisted in situ keratomileusis (LASIK) and other refractive procedures in which cataract surgical patients do not feel excluded by the wonders of modern corneal refractive results. The practice can become whole with common goals and expectations for all patients, with only a slight change in perception and the inclusion of techniques to control the 1 to 2 diopters of astigmatic or spherical error that is now the barrier to realization of this pleasant scenario. Refractive surgery can then encompass the spectrum of patients from the very young to the 60- and 70-year-old active seniors who have high expectations for quality of life and the benefits of reduced dependence on refractive correction. A good LASIK correction in a 30-year-old patient can be shared with his or her 65-year-old parent with similar results and a convergence of patient satisfaction.

This is the purpose of this book—to share the large and small approaches that we utilize in our practice and to make these techniques a reality for you in your own practice of refractive lens-based surgery.

Cataract Surgery: A Personal History

2

Richard C. Troutman, MD, FACS, FRCOphth

The operation for removal of the human cataract has been in evolution since its origins in antiquity. No matter what the approach to removal of the lens, it is still necessary to first penetrate or incise the globe in order to displace or remove the cataractous lens. When the surgery has restored a clear vision axis, the correction of the resulting aphakic hyperopia and the induced wound or naturally occurring astigmatism becomes essential to the final functional rehabilitation of the patient. Their refinement has been in progress for more than two centuries since Daviel first removed a cataract through an incision in the cornea in the late 17th century. My goal in this chapter is to give you a personal historical perspective on the evolution of the cataract operation during the past half-century as I have experienced it. I hope that you will find this an interesting and entertaining introduction.

The smallest incision still probably results from the couching procedure of ancient times. Though it is still performed today in some parts of the world, the complications from the retained displaced lens preclude its practical use. Since Daviel, the primary approach to removal of the human lens has been through an incision into the anterior chamber; and during most of the 19th century, the goal of cataract surgeons was to remove the lens through the smallest possible incision. This was facilitated by the extracapsular technique in which the lens was incised, allowed to mature, and soften before its partial removal. Additional procedures were often necessary to clear the visual axis to remove or incise the remaining lens and lens capsule. A sector iridectomy had to be performed to allow lens removal and avoid iris prolapse into the unsutured wound. In addition, multiple procedures had to be performed in minutes under topical anesthesia. When the visual axis had been finally cleared, the postoperative glare from the large pupil and lens remnants compromised the visual rehabilitation of the spectacle-corrected patient.

By the early 20th century, the necessity for several procedures as well as the severe complications from the extracapsular procedure and the long period necessary for recovery of vision led some surgeons to attempt removal of the lens in its capsule during a single procedure. Among the early advocates was Colonel Smith, an English surgeon practicing in India who reportedly used a fingernail to express the lens, the "Smith Indian" technique, while allowing the ash on his omnipresent cigar to grow to a phenomenal length. Another was Ignacio Barraquer, of Barcelona, Spain, the father of Joaquin and José, who removed the lens with a "ventosa," the prototype of the erisophake.

However, intracapsular lens extraction required a larger incision. As the incision was still left to heal by "first intention" without suture apposition, postoperative wound complications were frequent and a sector iridectomy was still considered a necessity. Nevertheless, cataract surgeons were reluctant to abandon the intracapsular method because of the advantages of the single procedure and, when successful, the more rapid rehabilitation. This and the continuing necessity to remove a sector of the iris led some surgeons in the decade before World War II to explore methods to better secure the cataract incision. By this time, local anesthesia included retrobulbar injection of novocaine to paralyze the extraocular muscles and lids, and akinesia, which could prevent involuntary movement of the eye and lids for up to 30 minutes. This gave surgeons the time to consider means for closing the wound.

I began my personal experience in this "revolution" in cataract surgery on April 1, 1945 when I entered training in ophthalmology at New York Hospital, Cornell Medical Center, Ithaca, NY. The head of our division, John M. McLean, was not only an outspoken advocate of intracapsular lens extraction, still not universally accepted, but also was recognized as the innovator of one of the best methods to close the cataract incision by preplacing edge-to-edge sutures in an intact globe. At the time it was virtually impossible to place the large-diameter, round, tapered needles then available in the opened eye without risking iris prolapse and lens expulsion that could be followed by vitreous, considered to be inviolate. As a result, most surgeons were using some form of preplaced sutures, inserted before the von Graefe knife or keratome and scissors incision.

The most commonly used preplaced sutures were overlying sutures. These were preplaced in a mattress fashion with one bite horizontal to the surgical limbus in the cornea and the second in the sclera distal to the limbus. The incision was made through the surgical limbus between the overlying loops. The track sutures (Voerhoeff) were preplaced in the cornea and sclera. At about half-thickness across the surgical limbus a large diameter 4-0 or 5-0 suture was being used. The cataract incision was made to cut through the sutures at their midpoint in the surgical limbus. The cut suture ends were withdrawn and the suture tracks rethreaded with a smaller diameter suture and needle in the opened eye.

The first method could cause inversion of the wound edges if drawn up too tightly or, at best, tenuous closure of the wound. The second left a window of opportunity for complications during the rethreading that was often difficult with no magnification. Many surgeons simply closed the wound by suturing the edge of the conjunctival flap to the distal conjunctiva. The sutures were so irritating that they had to be removed in a few days or weeks, leaving the wound to heal by "first intention." The result was a poorly healed incision that stretched over time to induce a flattening of the vertical meridian and often severe against-the-rule astigmatism.

While a resident at the Wilmer Institute in 1939, McLean devised a method to preplace an edge-to-edge suture in the cataract wound before the eye was opened. He made an 180-degree, partial penetrating incision vertically in the corneoscleral groove (surgical limbus) in the intact globe. He then passed the needle from cornea to sclera across the groove, leaving the 5-0 (later 6-0) braided silk suture exposed in its depth where it could be retrieved and looped out of the incision. The eye was then opened with a von Graefe knife—a survivor from the 19th century—that had been designed to make quick and accurate cataract incisions because of the severe time constraints inherent in the procedure (Figure 2-1). The long narrow blade was passed across the anterior chamber from one extremity of the groove to the opposite in the 180-degree meridian and then brought up to cut between the opened loop(s) of the sutures (usually two), hopefully leaving them intact.

The accurate completion of this incision was considered a rite of passage for residents. At

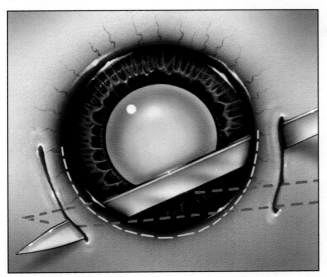

Figure 2-1. The von Graefe cataract incision.

worst, we could cut one or both of the two sutures, shave the iris, and even impale the lens in one fell swoop. Dr. McLean considered opening the eye with a keratome and cutting between the suture loops with a scissors (the other technique common at the time) to be beneath his dignity and, thus, ours. When all went well, the intact suture loops could be drawn up to securely close the eye to manage a threatened intraoperative complication and, as the lens was removed, without having to place sutures in the opened eye. The more secure closure usually permitted the preservation of the iris sphincter, "round pupil extraction," and prevented peripheral anterior synechia. The intact pupil eliminated the glare problem that had compromised postoperative vision for more than a century and served as a barrier to prevent vitreous incarceration in the wound meridian.

After the surgery, usually the older patients were kept in bed on their backs, their head movement restricted by sandbags, and they were kept bilaterally patched for a week or more. The suture knots were so irritating that the patients suffered constant tearing and they had to be removed 2 to 3 weeks after surgery, long before the wound was firmly healed. Spastic entropion frequently occurred, and the inverted lower lashes further contributed to the uncomfortable postoperative course. Some surgeons advocated using absorbable sutures for closure to avoid the necessity for removal. However, their dissolution time was unpredictable and when they failed to biodegrade they were even more difficult to remove. Although the incision was accurately apposed over the short-term, after suture removal the unsupported wound would stretch, sometimes even separate. This caused what I termed a "lambda-shaped incision profile," resulting in increasing flattening of the vertical meridian and inducing against-the-rule astigmatism. If the incision became partially separated and leaked aqueous, a flat anterior chamber would occur. The eye would become soft as the anterior chamber emptied. The choroid would detach, pushing the peripheral iris into the opened sections of the wound. If this did not reform the chamber, the vitreous would follow. Secondary glaucoma was the inevitable outcome, as well as chronic uveitis and retinal detachment.

It is unbelievable today to think that this chain of events was not attributed to poor wound closure but to some other mysterious cause. Hours of discussion were devoted to its etiology, but at the time few noticed that its disappearance as a complication coincided with microsurgical wound closure and, especially, the introduction of 10-0 nylon sutures.

The often significant postoperative astigmatism generated by the incision-induced flattening of the cornea was accepted as a "normal" accompaniment of cataract surgery. Even after successful cataract surgery, the usual aphakic spectacle correction could be more debilitating to the patient than his or her cataract had been. Though sclera-supported glass and methylmethacrylate contact lenses were becoming available, even when successfully fit they could be worn only a few hours at a time and were almost impossible for the usually older cataract patient to handle on a daily basis. Their lack of success was not due to poor wound healing and incision-induced astigmatic errors. McLean's professor and mentor at Wilmer, Dr. Alan Woods, published a widely read article in the *American Journal of Ophthalmology* on his trials in acclimating to aphakic spectacle vision, though he had successfully operated with the McLean technique. These compromising functional problems so preoccupied cataract surgeons that the refractive rehabilitation of the patient received little attention and aphakic correction remained much as it had been in the 19th century: relying primarily on spectacles.

Nevertheless, intracapsular cataract extraction was the state of the art from 1945 until well into the 1970s, and many cataract surgeons continued to use the preplaced McLean suture decades after I had given up its use. Such was its reputation that the Academy Course on this technique that he gave with two of his former fellow residents at Wilmer, Edward A. Maumenee and Jack S. Guyton, was "sold out" well in advance of the meeting for many years. I still consider myself most fortunate to have been under John's tutelage, as he was truly avant garde in the development of modern cataract surgery. In 1949, Dr. Bernard Samuels, a well-known ophthalmic pathologist, became like Lancelot in search of the Holy Grail when he tried to find a surgeon to perform an extracapsular extraction of his cataract. He had concluded from his study of pathologic aphakic eyes that a well-performed extracapsular operation was safer than intracapsular lens removal. He finally convinced his associate, Dr. Milton Berliner, whose textbook *Biomicroscopy of the Eye* was our bible, to perform the procedure—the outcome was never reported.

Anesthesia for Cataract Surgery

Another obstacle to accurate cataract incision and closure was anesthesia. Retrobulbar anesthesia and lid akinesia, as championed by Walter Atkinson, were only effective for about 30 minutes and was known as "local and vocal." General anesthesia was even less reliable. I recall Dr. Daniel Kirby, a famous cataract surgeon of the era, using the Flagg Can, manipulated by Dr. Flagg himself, for cataract anesthesia. This was a can of ether administered by "continuous drip" through a short length of tubing attached to a mask held over the patient's nose and mouth. If the eye survived the anesthesia, the postoperative nausea would challenge it again.

1949: Ridley's Intraocular Lens

In 1949, Dr. Harold Ridley, after an extracapsular cataract extraction, placed the first intraocular lens in the posterior chamber of an aphakic human eye in an attempt to restore the preoperative optics to their natural locus. It was made of Perspex (Imperial Chemical, London, England), a methylmethacrylate resin that he had found to be well-tolerated by the eye as a foreign body when shards were implanted accidentally from Spitfire windshields during the war. He reasoned that the physiologically positioned lens would resolve many of the optical problems inherent in spectacle correction. This intriguing idea prompted some surgeons to follow his example; however, severe complications and frequent lens dislocation in the early cases caused his technique to be abandoned. Even when the implant was temporarily retained, the power of the implanted lens was so grossly inaccurate that the optical results were disappointing. These many failures were due to poor incision and closure techniques but were overshadowed by the general view that this was a concept doomed to failure from the onset.

It was only a few years later that Strampelli began to implant his lens in the anterior chamber, where it could be more securely fixed in the iris sulcus as a secondary procedure after successful intracapsular cataract extraction. He also advocated implantation of his lens in phakic eyes for the correction of high myopia. The calculation of the individual implanted lens power was based on the preoperative refraction of the aphakic or highly myopic eye. However, with few exceptions, intraocular lenses could potentially correct only the spherical component and not the wound-induced astigmatism, as they still are today.

Zeiss Galilean Surgical Microscope

In 1951, during my senior residency, I had acquired and used a pair of binocular loupes that I felt helped me to better perform cataract incision and closure, as well as other anterior segment procedures. I preferred to sit rather than stand during surgery, which became yet another occasion for jest. An ear, nose, and throat colleague who had just begun to do middle ear surgery introduced by Shambaugh acquainted me with his Zeiss otologic microscope with six-step magnification up to 40x and allowed me to borrow it from his department. The same instrument was being used by gynecologists for diagnosis and management of cervical cancer but was soon abandoned after the Papinicalou technique became available. However, I found its inline binocular configuration and long working distance awkward for use in eye surgery.

In 1952 following the International Congress of Ophthalmology in New York, I went to Europe to visit clinics and see the work of some colleagues I had met there. Still in quest of a more suitable microscope for ophthalmic surgery, I visited the Zeiss factory in Oberkochen, Germany. While there, I met Dr. Hans Liffman, head of microscope development, and convinced him to modify the microscope that he had designed for use in otology and gynecology for ophthalmic surgery. Upon my suggestion, he angled the inline binoculars to 45 degrees, shortened the working distance to 200 mm, and modified the floor stand support so that I could use the microscope from a sitting position. The lateral positioning, tilting, focus, and magnification range were all manually adjusted. As I began to operate with the instrument, I thought about how these functions might be remotely controlled so that the surgeon would not have to move from the surgical field to make adjustments.

Microsurgery was only slowly accepted. One of our most prominent anterior segment surgeons and a pioneer in corneal surgery, Ramon Castroviejo, was proud to say he never used a microscope. Max Fine, another prominent corneal surgeon who stood about 5 feet 2 inches tall, remarked once after my lecture on the subject at the Chicago Ophthalmological Society that he was the only "true microsurgeon."

One reason for many surgeons' lack of interest in beginning to use the microscope was the necessity to change the magnification, which could cause loss of visualization at a critical time during the procedure. The floor stand was also somewhat unstable, requiring frequent manual repositioning of the field and refocusing. Eugene Cohen, an endocrinologist colleague, told me about a zoom microscope that was newly manufactured by Bausch & Lomb (Claremont, Calif), which he was using for his dissections of rat adrenals. I reasoned that continuous visualization through the range of magnification would eliminate the "blind spots" of the Zeiss Galilean system and that this might be enhanced if one could remotely change the magnification. At the American Academy of Ophthalmology meeting that year, I took my idea to the Keeler Instrument Company (London, England), whom I knew through their intraocular lens division. They were able to build the Bausch & Lomb microscope with a reversing motor control so that I could change the magnification by a two-position foot control. To better stabilize the patient's eye under the microscope, Keeler used a headrest designed by Mr. Dermot Pierse, an ophthalmic surgeon from Birmingham England. I had the headrest mounted on a vertically adjustable hydraulic floor support, which maintained the operative field in stable relationship to the microscope, requiring only minimal manual focusing. For its time this instrument was widely distributed. I saw one being used when I visited Moscow some 15 years later.

10-0 Nylon Sutures

In 1962, I was introduced to a new 10-0 nylon suture material by Gunter Mackensen and Heinrich Harms of Tubingen, Germany, which they were using to close cataract and keratoplasty incisions. Once placed, tied, and the knot buried, the suture loops remained inert in the tissues and could be left in place for as long as necessary to securely hold the wound until firmly healed. They had obtained the material from a tire manufacturer and had wound it on small bobbins. They gave me enough thread to last for years. They placed the sutures with 5-mm eyed needles from Klein (Heidelberg, Germany), which I also brought back with me. The nylon thread was so fine that it was necessary for my surgical nurse to use the microscope to thread it to the needles. 10-0 nylon was a true microsurgery suture, impossible to see, let alone use, effectively without magnification. We soon learned that the suture could not be removed in 4 to 6 weeks as we had done with virgin silk. However, if left in place for 3 to 6 months, more physiologic healing took place without the scarring we had seen with silk and catgut sutures. If we took care to bury the knots as Mackensen had advised, patients were comfortable from the day of surgery on. Immediate postoperative astigmatism was now largely suture-induced and the wound-induced component became evident only when the sutures were removed. As I later discovered and published, this material could be used safely with through-and-through bites that closed the corneal incision from back to front. The resulting full thickness healed against-the-rule astigmatic shift from the lambda-shaped scar of superficial corneal incision closure. Nylon's consistency and elasticity made possible the use of "slip knots" that could be more accurately tensioned during wound closure.

3 Incision Wound Healing

Paul Ernest, MD

Introduction

Sutureless incisions for cataract surgery should ideally remain sealed with increased intraocular pressure and be able to withstand increased external pressure to the posterior aspect. Cadaver eye studies have shown that meeting these criteria requires an internal corneal lip of at least 1.5 mm and a square wound. Scleral incisions can meet these criteria but sacrifice aesthetics and surgical efficiency. Clear corneal incisions provide aesthetics and surgical efficiency but less wound stability. An ideal incision would combine scleral incision stability with the aesthetics and efficiency of the clear corneal incision.

An incision at the limbus was tested to assess its ability to meet these criteria. The incision originated at the limbus, gaining about 0.5 mm in tunnel length over a clear corneal incision—enough to obtain a nearly square profile of 3 mm in width and 2.5 to 3.0 mm in length, while providing the aesthetics and surgical efficiency of a clear corneal incision. Each was tested in stepped, paracentesis, and hinged profile, using the methods of previous studies. The hinged outperformed the stepped, which was inturn superior to the paracentesis. For all types, limbal outperformed corneal, even when the limbal and clear corneal incisions were equally rectangular—evidence that the limbus provides added stability. Thus, the limbal incision is equal to the clear corneal incision in aesthetics and surgical efficiency, slightly superior in patient comfort, and far more stable than a clear corneal incision.

Historical Perspective

In 1972, when I started my training in ophthalmology, all cataract incisions started in the limbal area. They were short, beveled incisions requiring suture closure. In 1977, Dr. Richard Kratz introduced the concept of the scleral tunnel incision. This is a two-plane incision, starting approximately 2 mm behind the posterior aspect of the surgical limbus. The anterior chamber was entered in the area of the iris root: 10-0 nylon sutures—interrupted or shoestring closure—were used to secure the wound. The advantage of the scleral tunnel incision was to reduce the induced astigmatism that sutures caused on the corneal curvature by hav-

Figure 3-1. A 4-mm incision with peripheral anterior synechiae.

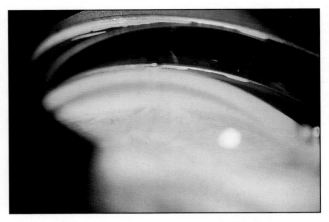

Figure 3-2. A persistent filtering bleb subsequent to the peripheral anterior synechiae.

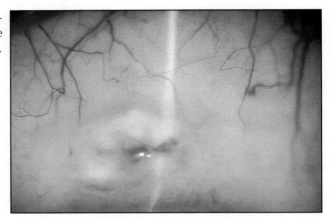

ing the sutures more posteriorly placed.[1] Problems with the scleral tunnel incision included hyphemas due to bleeding within the scleral tunnel and delayed filtering blebs due to peripheral anterior synechiae internally, acting as a wick[2] (Figures 3-1 and 3-2).

Era of Foldable Lenses and "One-Stitch" Suture Closure

In October 1989, the first foldable intraocular lens gained US Food and Drug Administration (FDA) approval. The AMO SI 18 from Allergan (Irvine, Calif) is a silicone lens with polypropylene haptics (Figure 3-3). With the use of folding devices (ie, McDonald-Katina), the lens could be inserted through an incision of 4 mm. Surgeons found that closing the wound with a single suture resulted in greater wound stability and faster visual rehabilitation. Glasses could be dispensed in 4 weeks' time[3] (Figures 3-4 to 3-11).

Dr. John Shepard of Las Vegas, Nev improved on the single-stitch closure, introducing the horizontal mattress closure in which the roof was attached to the floor of the tunnel incision with a horizontal 10-0 nylon suture, leaving a small gap in the external aspect of the

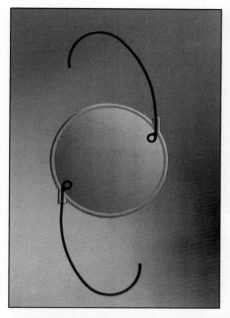

Figure 3-3. Allergan AMO SI 18 NGB intraocular lens.

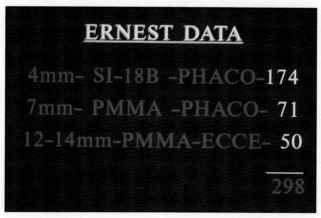

ERNEST DATA

4mm– SI-18B –PHACO-174

7mm– PMMA –PHACO– 71

12-14mm-PMMA-ECCE– 50

298

Figure 3-4. Demographics of a study comparing 4 mm, 7 mm, and 14 mm incisions.

incision. The horizontal suture closure allowed for even greater wound stability and less induced with-the-rule astigmatism and glasses could be dispensed in 1 to 2 weeks' time post-surgery.[4]

In spite of this wonderful technology and enhanced visual rehabilitation, hyphemas and delayed filtering blebs still plagued the ophthalmic surgeons.

Era of Sutureless Cataract Surgery

In January 1990, Dr. Michael McFarland of Pine Bluff, Ark hypothesized that the suture was the source of the bleeding in the scleral tunnel which resulted in delayed hyphema 1 to 2 days postsurgery. Dr. McFarland wished to create an incision that required no sutures. He

Figure 3-5. Demographics of a study comparing 4 mm, 7 mm, and 14 mm incisions.

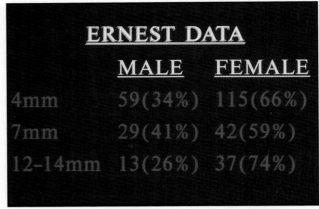

Figure 3-6. Data at 1 to 3 months.

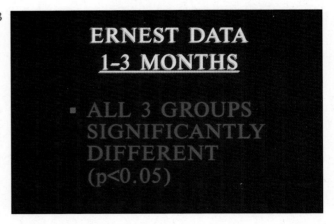

Figure 3-7. Data at 1 to 3 months.

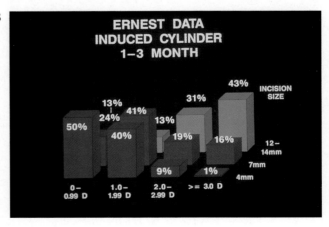

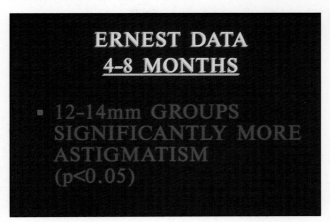

Figure 3-8. Data at 4 to 8 months.

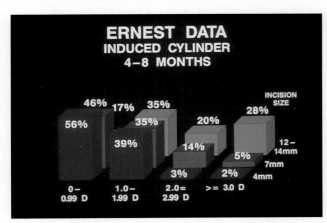

Figure 3-9. Data at 4 to 8 months.

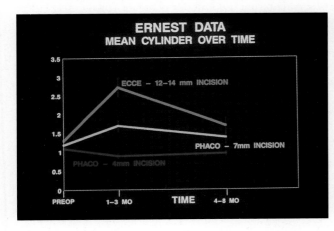

Figure 3-10. Wound stability over time.

Figure 3-11. Wound stability over time.

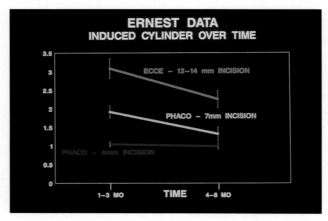

hypothesized making a long scleral tunnel incision that was a "funnel incision," in which the internal aspect was wider than the external aspect. He envisioned the internal aspect of 4 to 4.5 mm and the external aspect of 3.0 mm. He created vertical cuts in the floor of the incision near the external aspect to allow relaxation and passage of the intraocular lens. The incision was approximately 4 mm posterior to the posterior aspect of the surgical limbus (see Figure 3-11).

The Internal Corneal Lip

I was present at a meeting in Phoenix, Ariz when Dr. McFarland introduced his idea of sutureless surgery in January 1990. At that time, I had been working on the problem of hyphemas and delayed filtering blebs and felt that if the incision was carried into the cornea, creating an internal corneal lip; the intraocular pressure would seal the wound internally, thereby preventing blood products from entering the anterior chamber (Figure 3-12). The corneal lip would also prevent delayed filtering blebs by preventing egress of fluid from the anterior chamber due to peripheral anterior synechiae (Figures 3-13 and 3-14). When Dr. McFarland introduced the idea of sutureless cataract surgery, I felt the internal corneal lip would be an added advantage to his long scleral tunnel and proceeded in February 1980 to use Dr. McFarland's scleral tunnel concept along with my concept of the internal corneal lip (Figure 3-15).

I found the surgery to be very cumbersome and difficult. I felt that there was tremendous oarlocking, as well as poor visualization. The risk for complications seemed significant. On February 20, 1990, I moved the incision more anterior to approximately 3 mm behind the surgical limbus. I made the incision 4.0 mm in width, eliminating the need to use the cuts in the scleral tunnel floor. I maintained an internal corneal lip of 1.5 mm. The wounds were extremely secure. Patients were brought to Wayne State University Kresge Eye Institute for grand rounds presentation of February 28, 1990.

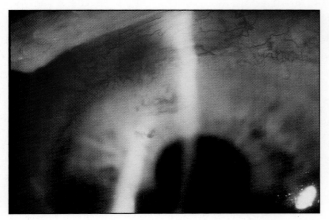

Figure 3-12. Blood products stopped by the internal corneal lip incision.

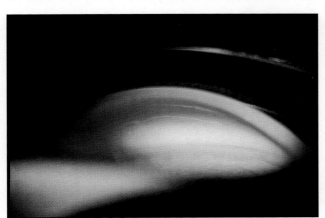

Figure 3-13. A gonioscopic view of the internal corneal lip incision.

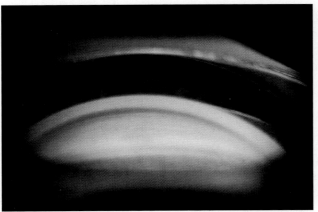

Figure 3-14. A 1-day postoperative gonioscopy of the internal corneal lip incision surrounded by blood products.

Figure 3-15. A histologic section of the incision, demonstrating internal corneal lip.

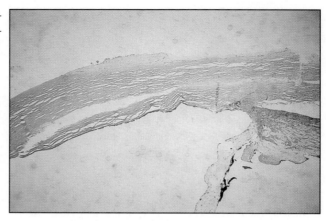

Modification of Wound Architecture Based on Scientific Experiments

1990 Cadaver Eye Study

In the Spring of 1990, a cadaver model was used to test the stability of wounds with and without internal corneal lips and with and without various suture closures. It was found that the internal corneal lip allowed considerable resistance to a rise in intraocular pressure.[5] A sutureless wound with an internal corneal lip gave a significant resistance to wound leak with rise in intraocular pressure compared to wounds that did not have internal corneal lips that were closed with radial or horizontal suture closures. Only a wound of 4 mm in width with a horizontal suture closure performed well with a rise in intraocular pressure.[6]

The advantages of the internal corneal lip were also proven clinically:

1. Patients having expulsive choroidal hemorrhage could be dealt with appropriately. By removing instrumentation, a sealed incision is created and the expulsive hemorrhage can be dealt with.

2. Patients with significant respiratory and cardiac distress at the time of surgery could be managed by removing instrumentation, having an immediate seal of the wound, addressing the patient's medical needs, and returning at an appropriate time for continuation of the surgery.

3. Postoperatively, many anecdotal incidents were noted in which patients had trauma to the eye, either by falling on their face or being struck in the eye, resulting in no dehiscence of the cataract wound.

Gonioscopy Study

One hundred and six patients undergoing different types of cataract incisions were evaluated using gonioscopy. The wounds were 11 mm, 7 mm, and 4 mm. The 4-mm incisions were subdivided into two groups: those without a corneal lip and those with a corneal lip.[6]

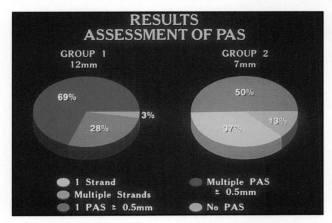

Figure 3-16. Results of a gonioscopy study comparing 12 mm and 7 mm incisions without corneal lip.

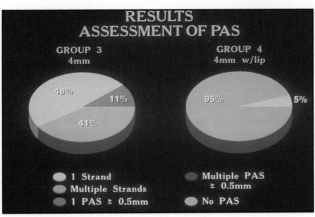

Figure 3-17. Results of a gonioscopy study comparing 4 mm incisions without corneal lip and a 4 mm incision with corneal lip.

Evaluation with gonioscopy revealed either band-like peripheral anterior synechiae (multiple or single), strand-like peripheral anterior synechiae (multiple or single), and no peripheral anterior synechiae. In patients with 11-mm incisions, 100% of the patients had peripheral anterior synechiae and most of the patients had band-like formation. With 7-mm incisions, the majority of the patients had peripheral anterior synechiae that were a combination of band- and strand-like. With 4-mm incisions without a corneal lip, there was still evidence of peripheral anterior synechiae in 59% of patients. Patients with band-like peripheral anterior synechiae also were found to have delayed filtering blebs. In patients with the internal corneal lip, only one patient out of 20 (5%) had an isolated strand of peripheral anterior synechiae (Figures 3-16 through 3-19). None of the patients had delayed filtering blebs.

Gonioscopy confirmed that the trabecular meshwork was left untouched following cataract surgery in patients with an internal corneal lip, leaving it available for argon laser trabeculoplasty in patients with chronic open-angle glaucoma.

Figure 3-18. Demographics of a gonioscopy study.

RESULTS ASSESSMENT OF PAS				
	GROUP 1 12mm		GROUP 2 7mm	
	n	%	n	%
Total patients	29	100%	30	100%
Patients with PAS	29	100%	26	87%
1 Isolated Strand	0	-	11	37%
Multiple Isolated Strands	1	3%	0	-
1 PAS ≥ 0.5mm	8	28%	15	50%
Multiple PAS ≥ 0.5mm	20	69%	0	-

Figure 3-19. Demographics of a gonioscopy study.

RESULTS ASSESSMENT OF PAS				
	GROUP 3 4mm		GROUP 4 4mm w/lip	
	n	%	n	%
Total patients	27	100%	20	100%
Patients with PAS	16	59%	1	5%
1 Isolated Strand	13	48%	1	5%
Multiple Isolated Strands	0	-	0	-
1 PAS ≥ 0.5mm	3	11%	0	-
Multiple PAS ≥ 0.5mm	0	-	0	-

1991 Cadaver Eye Study

In 1991, a second study using cadaver models was performed, evaluating the question of "what is the ideal amount of internal corneal lip necessary to give the best wound stability?"[6] Geometry of the incision was also studied. Four conclusions were observed:

1. Internal corneal lip of 1.5 mm gave the best resistance to deformation pressure. Similar wounds with internal corneal lips less than 1.5 mm showed less resistance to deformation pressure (Figure 3-20).

2. Narrower incisions did better than wider incisions. Four-millimeter incisions performed better than 5-mm incisions and a 6-mm incision with the same amount of internal corneal lip in all incisions (Figure 3-21).

3. Square wounds, in which the width of the incision and the overall length including that of the 1.5-mm internal corneal lip, gave the best resistance to deformation pressure. In fact, deformation pressure of 525 PSI found no evidence of wound leak in 4.0-mm square incisions with a 1.5-mm internal corneal lip.

4. Nonsquare wounds with increased IOP resisted deformation pressure better than the same wound constuction with normal IOP (Figure 3-22).

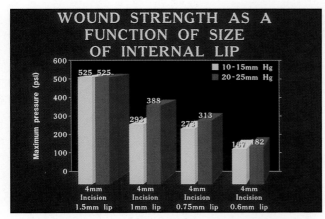

Figure 3-20. Effect of internal corneal lip with the same width incision and essentially the same length. This demonstrates effectiveness of the 1.5 mm internal corneal lip.

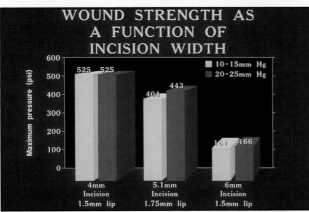

Figure 3-21. Comparison between 4 mm incision, 5.1 mm incision, and the relatively same internal corneal lip.

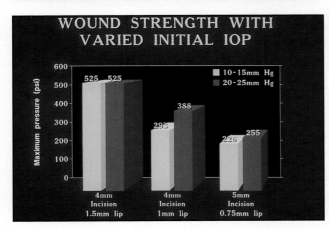

Figure 3-22. The effectiveness of intraocular pressure on incisions that leak.

From these studies using scleral corneal incisions, we recommended that a 4-mm square wound with a 1.5-mm internal corneal lip was the best designed incision with the technology available for intraocular lens implantation in 1991.

Introduction of Sutureless Corneal Incisions

1991 Cadaver Eye Study

In the Spring of 1992 in San Diego, Calif, Dr. Howard Fine introduced a sutureless corneal incision. He derived this idea when visiting Dr. Kimiya Shimizu in Tokyo, Japan in the Fall of 1991. Dr. Shimizu had been using clear corneal incisions with a suture since 1989. Dr. Fine improved on the technique and introduced the sutureless version of the clear corneal incision. The original corneal incisions were a minimum of 4 mm in width due to implant technology and 1.75 mm in length. European surgeons used clear corneal incisions of 5.25 to 5.50 mm in width with the same 1.75 mm in length.

These incisions were performed at the temporal aspect. Aesthetically, the eyes had an "untouched" appearance postoperatively. Surgical efficiency improved tremendously. Dr. Mannus Kraft found that at least 2 minutes in time could be saved by performing this type of surgery using the temporal approach.

There was tremendous concern regarding wound stability of corneal incisions. These incisions were obviously nonsquare. If the corneal tissue was stretched, it did not return to its original configuration. There were anecdotal incidences of endophthalmitis. Presentations at subsequent ASCRS meetings demonstrated incidences of endophthalmitis in patients with these types of incisions.[7]

A cadaver study by my colleagues and myself evaluated clear corneal incisions relative to scleral corneal incisions.[6] Again, we found that the geometry of the incision was key. A square corneal incision, whether it be 1 x 1, 2 x 2, 3 x 3, or 3.2 x 3.2, gave the same stability as a square scleral corneal incision with a 1.5-mm corneal component (Table 3-1). The difficulty in performing cataract surgery through a 1-mm or 2-mm square corneal incision was obvious. Technology was not available to allow surgical removal of the lens or implantation of the substitute lens. The 3.2-mm square clear corneal incision could be performed, but the encroachment on the visual axis made this technique undesirable.

The cadaver study also showed that wound stability was influenced by two factors: 1.) the geometry and 2.) the intraocular pressure. A change in tunnel length from a 2-mm tunnel to a 2.5-mm with an incision width of 3.2 mm gave eight times resistance to deformation pressure at normal intraocular pressure settings of 10 to 15 mmHg. Going from an intraocular pressure of 10 to 15 mmHg to that of 20 to 25 mmHg with the same 3.2 x 2.0 mm incision clear cornea also gave eight to 10 times improvement in resistance to deformation pressure. It was recommended that if nonsquare or rectangular corneal incisions were to be used, it was important to keep the intraocular pressure elevated at the end of the procedure (Table 3-2).

Table 3-1

Pressure Applied Posterior to Incision:
Square Wounds Only

Observations
- Results with wounds of 3.2 mm or less are similar to results with 4.0 mm square wounds
- Wounds withstood maximum pressure of 525 psi with no leaks

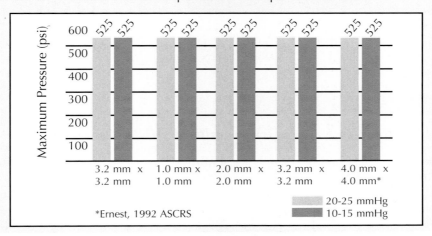

*Ernest, 1992 ASCRS

Table 3-2

Pressure Applied Posterior to Incision

Incision	Maximum External Pressure	
	IOP 10 to 15 mmHg	IOP 20 to 25 mmHg
SC 3.2 mm x 3.2 mm	525 psi, no leaks	525 psi, no leaks
CC 3.2 mm x 3.2 mm	525 psi, no leaks	525 psi, no leaks
CC 2.0 mm x 2.0 mm	525 psi, no leaks	525 psi, no leaks
CC 1.0 mm x 1.0 mm	525 psi, no leaks	525 psi, no leaks
CC 3.2 mm x 2.5 mm	101 psi, iris prolapse	187 psi, iris prolapse
CC 3.2 mm x 2.0 mm	13 psi, iris prolapse	114 psi, iris prolapse

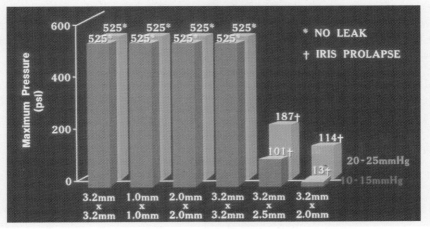

Table 3-3

Pressure at Incision Failure 10 to 15 mmHg

Incision Width	Corneal Paracentesis	Limbal Paracentesis	Stepped	Hinged
2.5 mm	54.6	124.4	93.5	120.8
3.0 mm	45.2	112.9	62.0	91.9
3.5 mm	32.6	55.6	61.4	88.7
4.0 mm	< 10	21.5	21.0	44.6
4.5 mm	< 10	11.6	< 10	11.6
5.0 mm	< 10	< 10	< 10	< 10

Table 3-4

Pressure at Incision Failure 20 to 25 mmHg

Incision Width	Corneal Paracentesis	Limbal Paracentesis	Stepped	Hinged
2.5 mm	121.3	263.6	108.2	199.0
3.0 mm	91.9	134.4	84.0	134.9
3.5 mm	65.1	98.7	69.8	125.5
4.0 mm	33.6	53.6	31.5	70.4
4.5 mm	< 10	23.1	10.5	43.1
5.0 mm	< 10	< 10	< 10	< 10

1993 Cadaver Eye Study

With the popularity of nonsquare corneal incisions, a study was performed to see if there was a critical width where these incisions could be predictable and more stable. Comparison was made between three corneal incisions: 1.) a paracentesis, 2.) a stepped, and 3.) a hinged incision, as described by Dr. David Langerman of Orangeburg, NY. It was found that at either low or moderate intraocular pressure settings, a 3.0-mm width was the critical width for a corneal paracentesis incision. A 3.5-mm width was the critical width for a corneal stepped or hinged incision. Any incision greater than these measurements would result in significant lack of wound stability[7] (Tables 3-3 and 3-4).

In 1993, the technology for implantation of intraocular lenses through a 3 mm incision had not been readily achieved. Question: Could an incision be made that gave all the advantages of a corneal incision—namely aesthetics and efficiency of surgery—still use a temporal approach, use of topical anesthesia, and still have the stability of qualities of a square wound, decreased foreign body sensation, ability to stretch the tissue, and be very reproducible? Could such an incision be made? It was time to re-evaluate the area of the limbus.

Table 3-5

Unpaired T-Test for Pressure Grouping Variable Technique: Hypothesized Difference

	Mean Difference	DF	T-Value	P-Value
CC, LB	-0.319	22	-3.278	0.0034

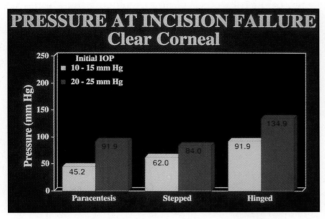

Figure 3-23. The relative strength to deformation pressure on corneal versus limbal comparing paracentesis, stepped, and hinged at intraocular pressure settings of 10 to 15 mmHg and 20 to 25 mmHg.

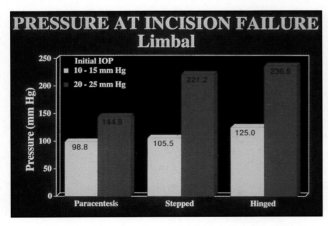

Figure 3-24. The relative strength to deformation pressure on corneal versus limbal comparing paracentesis, stepped, and hinged at intraocular pressure settings of 10 to 15 mmHg and 20 to 25 mmHg.

1994 Cadaver Eye Study

A cadaver eye study in 1994 evaluated nonsquare incisions that were 3.0 mm in width and 1.75 mm in tunnel length, with the only variable being that of location. Paracentesis, stepped, and hinged incisions were all made both 0.5 mm into clear cornea and at the limbal area. Intraocular pressures were kept to 10 to 15 mmHg and 20 to 25 mmHg, respectively, for each group of incisions[6] (Table 3-5 and Figures 3-23 and 3-24).

Results showed a paracentesis incision that started at the limbus gave 50% to 100% resistance in deformation pressure compared to the same incision started 0.5 mm into clear cornea. The hinged incision gave a 30% to 50% greater resistance to deformation pressure when starting at the limbus compared to starting in corneal tissue. Explanation: it is known that limbal tissue has elastic fibers, which allow the tissue to be stretched. It is believed that these elastic fibers play a role in the resistance to deformation pressure.

Critics of Cadaver Eye Studies

Critics of cadaver eye studies claim that cadaver studies do not give an accurate picture of wound stability because of a physiologic mechanism called the endothelial pump. Critics hypothesize that the endothelial pump, through its mechanism of removing fluid from the incision, causes a suction-like seal of the incision. Video demonstrations were given at meetings that showed proof of the endothelial pump theory. A "finger test" was done to push on wounds, demonstrating that they did not leak due to this endothelial pump mechanism. The only problem with the demonstration was that the intraocular pressures were not standardized and, in fact, it was clearly evident through these demonstrations that the intraocular pressure was elevated due to the posterior displacement of the iris lens diaphragm. Finger tests were only done on 3.0-mm corneal paracentesis incisions. Finger tests on 3.5-mm corneal paracentesis incisions showed a leak.

Work of Carlos DeFigueiredo, MD, Sao Paolo, Brazil

Dr. DeFigueiredo performed work on a living rabbit model, evaluating three types of corneal incisions: paracentesis, hinged, and square. All incisions were made with diamond knives, no deformation of the incision was performed through instrumentation. Stromal hydration was used in all three incisions. Dr. DeFigueiredo found that 15 minutes poststromal hydration, the cornea was clear of any stromal edema, indicating that the endothelial pump was effective in removing all fluid within 15 minutes. Within 5 minutes upon removal of the fluid, he performed deformation tests. He found that the paracentesis incision leaked with 5 grams of weight, the hinged incision leaked with 40 grams of weight, and the square corneal incision showed minimal leak with 100 grams of weight. Dr. DeFigueiredo concluded that the endothelial pump was only effective in removing fluid, and was not effective in wound stability. He was very concerned about the stability of the paracentesis corneal incision and even recommended that this type of corneal incision should be sutured or glued.[8]

Work of Richard Tipperman, MD, Wills Eye Hospital, Philadelphia

A study was performed at Wills Eye Hospital with Dr. Tipperman and myself in January 1996 using a living feline model. Paracentesis incisions of 3.0 mm in width, 1.75 mm in length were performed in each eye of the cat. The incision in the right eye started in clear cornea and the left eye at the limbus. There was no distortion of the wound through instrumentation. There was no stromal hydration.

On the first postoperative day, Dr. Tipperman noticed a fibrinous exudate in all 18 right eyes with clear corneal incisions. He believed that this was due to the hypotony that stems from a corneal incision without reformation of the anterior chamber and without stromal hydration. In the left eyes with the limbal incisions, none of the 18 eyes revealed the exudate.[9]

Deformation studies were then performed at the 24-hour postoperative mark (see Figure 3-17). The findings of this study correlated beautifully with the 1994 cadaver study, demonstrating again that the endothelial pump was not a factor in wound stability.

University of Berlin, Germany, Department of Ophthalmology Study

In 1995, the Department of Ophthalmology at the University of Berlin published a study in which 188 human eyes were tested postsurgery.[9] All eyes had nonsquare, rectangular incisions. The location of the incisions were both superior and temporal. The incisions were scleral cornea or limbal cornea. Deformation pressure studies were performed at 1 day postsurgery and 1 week postsurgery.

Results: using human eyes, all rectangular wounds leaked 1 day postsurgery. However, at 7 days postsurgery, all wounds were completely sealed regardless of superior versus temporal location.

The Descemet Bond

There have been occasions when surgeons had to re-enter an eye due to a decentration of a foldable intraocular lens. These eyes had scleral corneal incisions. Observers, including myself, found that it was easy to find the plane of the scleral tunnel. Dissection into the cornea was also easily done; however, there was an apparent bond at Descemet's membrane, making it very difficult to enter the anterior chamber. A keratome blade had to be reinserted to break the bond of Descemet's membrane.

Avascular versus Vascular Origin of Incision

In addition to geometry and construction, is there a difference in the healing process of an incision whether one starts in an avascular (clear corneal) incision or a vascular (limbal or scleral) incision? Studies at Wills Eye Hospital and Kresge Eye Institute were performed to evaluate this question.[9]

Animal studies were performed at Wills Eye Hospital and Kresge Eye Institute using a feline model. Dr. Chris Kardassis performed a fellow eye study using a paracentesis incision of 3.0 x 1.75 mm in which the right eye was a clear corneal incision and the left eye was a limbal incision. He tested the resistance to deformation pressure at days 4 through 11 (Figure 3-25). Looking at the graph of the limbal incision, one notes that at day 6, there is considerable resistance of deformation pressure that maintains itself through day 11. This corresponds nicely to the clinical findings of the University of Berlin, where they found that

Figure 3-25. The results of pressure testing on the feline model, comparing clear corneas and limbal incisions.

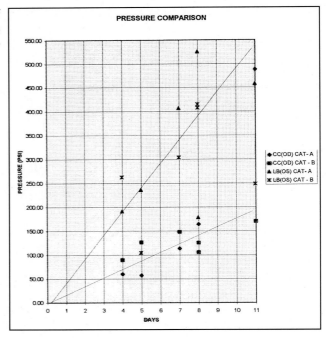

wounds with vascular origin were completely sealed in 7 days. The corneal incision, however, did not achieve these levels through the 11-day test period. A nonpaired T-test analysis was performed to see if there was a statistical significance between the limbal and corneal incisions. It was found to be highly statistically significant with a P-value of 0.0034 (see Table 3-5).

Histologic Evaluation

Dr. Richard Tipperman and Dr. Ralph Eagle of Wills Eye Hospital histologically evaluated the healing process of the feline incisions at 1 week, 1 month, and 2 months. The selected eyes did not undergo any deformation pressure studies. There were strictly paracentesis incisions without any manipulation of the wound intraoperatively or postoperatively.

Findings: at 1 week post-surgery on histologic evaluation, there was no healing of the corneal incision at all (Figure 3-26). Anterior limbal incisions showed a fibroblastic response, which completely sealed the wound 7 days post-surgery (Figure 3-27). If the incision was made to the mid and posterior limbus, the fibroblastic response was greater and, again, the wound was completely sealed in 7 days (Figure 3-28). These findings correlated beautifully with the deformation pressure studies of Dr. Kardassis, as well as the clinical findings of the University of Berlin on human eyes. This also demonstrates the concern on the part of many surgeons regarding corneal incisions in an avascular origin as to the stability of these wounds and their safety in various activities.

At 1 month postsurgery, the corneal incision again demonstrated no healing. At 2 months postsurgery, the corneal incision did heal through a fibroblastic response (Figure 3-

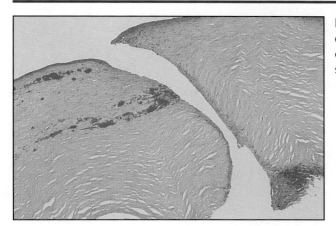

Figure 3-26. A histologic slide of a 1-week postoperative clear corneal incision demonstrating no healing.

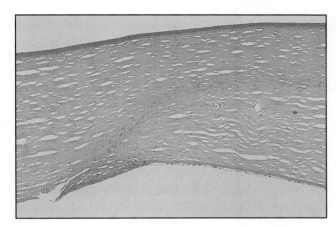

Figure 3-27. An anterior limbal incision showing fibroblastic response with complete healing at 7 days postoperatively.

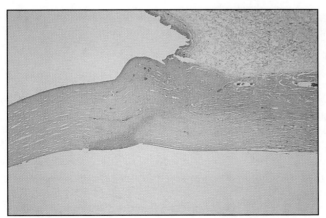

Figure 3-28. A mid to posterior limbal incision 7 days postoperatively with complete healing of the incision.

Figure 3-29. A clear corneal incision 60 days postoperatively with a fibroblastic response and complete healing of the incision.

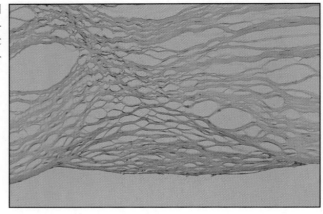

29). The appearance of the limbal incision at 2 months was identical to that of the limbal incision at 1 week postsurgery.

Discussion of Findings

Avascular versus Vascular

Both the corneal and limbal incisions healed through a fibroblastic response. The origin for the fibroblastic response of limbal incisions is probably vascular; however, the possibility of stem cell differentiation cannot be ruled out. The origin of the fibroblastric response for corneal incisions is similar to that of a corneal transplant. The apposition of stromal keratocytes and the transformation of stromal keratocytes to fibroblasts is the suggested mechanism. The significance, however, is the timing of the response. The fibroblastic response for avascular origin is 7 days, compared to 60 days for the avascular clear corneal incision.

Induced Astigmatism With Limbal Incisions

Evaluation was made of the 3.2 mm limbal incision based on vector analysis using a superior and temporal approach. Evaluation of uncorrected vision at 1 day postsurgery and corrected vision at 2 weeks postsurgery was also evaluated. Did the early fibroblastic response give any adverse effect on the induced astigmatism of these incisions?

A retrospective study looking at 599 patients was performed.[9] The study was conducted by independent observers who pulled 599 charts randomly. Demographics and breakdown of patients regarding age and location of the incision are described (see Figures 3-18 and 3-19).

Results: findings of the study show there was no statistical difference between the uncorrected vision of a superior versus temporal approach, using a limbal incision at 1 day postsurgery. This contradicts previous findings, and impressions by myself and others that the uncorrected visual acuity with the temporal approach is better 1 day postsurgery than superior approach. Vector analysis of Jaffe also shows no statistical difference between a superior

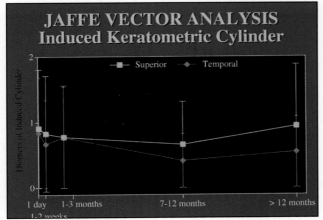

Figure 3-30. The vector analysis of Jaffe demonstrating temporal and superior limbal incisions with a 4-mm scleral corneal incision as a standard.

Figure 3-31. The vector analysis of Jaffe demonstrating temporal and superior limbal incisions with a 4-mm scleral corneal incision as a standard.

JAFFE VECTOR ANALYSIS
Induced Keratometric Cylinder

	1 day	1-2 wks	1-3 mos	7-12 mos	>12 mos
Superior					
Mean	0.91	0.83	0.78	0.66	0.94
S.D.	(±0.90)	(±0.88)	(±0.84)	(±0.73)	(±1.01)
N	355	267	158	26*	34*
Temporal					
Mean	0.84	0.67	0.77	0.41	0.54
S.D.	(±0.63)	(±0.58)	(±0.75)	(±0.26)	(±0.50)
N	239	193	86	13*	30*

* small sample size

and temporal approach with induced astigmatism (Figures 3-30 and 3-31). Cravey analysis also reveals minimal change in the axis using a limbal incision (Figures 3-32 and 3-33). Corneal topography is pre- and post-surgery for a limbal incision of 3.2 mm also shows minimal flattening (Figures 3-34 and 3-35).

Work of Dr. Rupert Menapace, Vienna, Austria

Dr. Menapace evaluated various incision sites and locations through corneal topography (Figure 3-36). He looked for changes in the corneal topography based on the incision at 1 week, 1 month, 2 months, and 3 months postsurgery. Dr. Menapace found that a square wound 4 mm in width with a 1.5-mm corneal lip gave minimal to no corneal topography changes (Figure 3-37). He found that the clear corneal paracentesis incision 3 mm wide also gave minimal to no corneal topography changes (Figure 3-38). However, if the corneal incision was larger than 3.0 mm, there were significant induced corneal topography changes.

Figure 3-32. The Cravey analysis of temporal versus superior limbal incisions with a 4-mm scleral corneal incision as a standard.

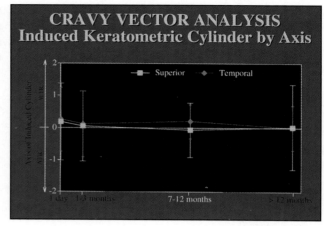

Figure 3-33. The Cravey analysis of temporal versus superior limbal incisions with a 4-mm scleral corneal incision as a standard.

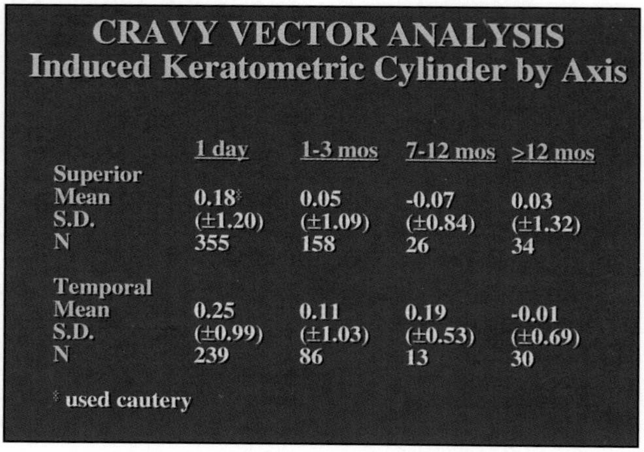

CRAVY VECTOR ANALYSIS
Induced Keratometric Cylinder by Axis

	1 day	1-3 mos	7-12 mos	≥12 mos
Superior				
Mean	0.18*	0.05	-0.07	0.03
S.D.	(±1.20)	(±1.09)	(±0.84)	(±1.32)
N	355	158	26	34
Temporal				
Mean	0.25	0.11	0.19	-0.01
S.D.	(±0.99)	(±1.03)	(±0.53)	(±0.69)
N	239	86	13	30

* used cautery

Figure 3-34. Preoperative and 1-day postoperative corneal topography results of a temporal limbal cataract incision.

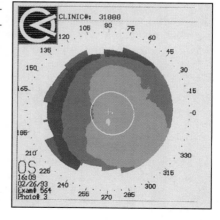

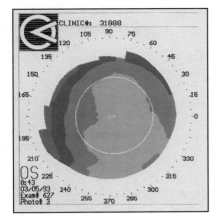

Figure 3-35. Preoperative and 1-day postoperative corneal topography results of a temporal limbal cataract incision.

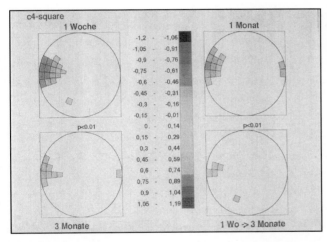

Figure 3-36. Incision sites and locations through corneal topography.

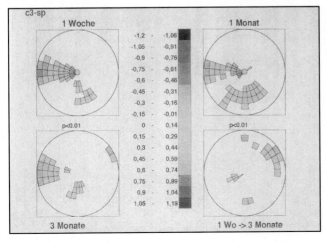

Figure 3-37. Incision sites and locations through corneal topography.

Figure 3-38. Topography changes.

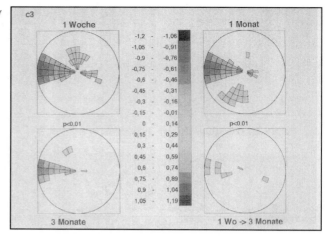

Figure 3-39. Incisions made in the sclera.

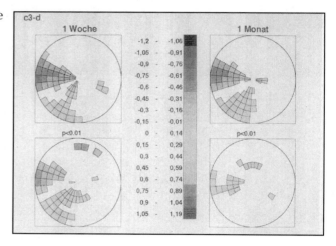

Dr. Menapace concluded that paracentesis incisions of 3 mm starting in the cornea or at the limbus would give similar results regarding corneal topography. This also corresponded beautifully to the cadaver study of 1993 showing the 3-mm critical width and wound stability for paracentesis incisions. Dr. Menapace felt that if an incision was 3.2 to 4 mm, the incision should be made in the anterior to posterior limbal region. Incisions 4 mm and greater should be made in the sclera (Figures 3-39 and 3-40).

Full Circle

It is interesting that since 1972 when I was introduced to cataract surgery starting at the limbal area that we as surgeons have tended to go full circle (Figure 3-41). We went back to the sclera in 1987. We used the corneal lip component in 1990 to begin the era of sutureless surgery. We advanced into the cornea in 1992 and now surgeons have moved back to the anterior limbus from an area of clear cornea, and those in the sclera have moved up more into the limbal area.

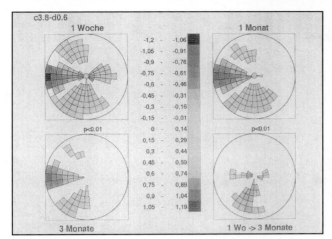

Figure 3-40. Incisions made in the sclera.

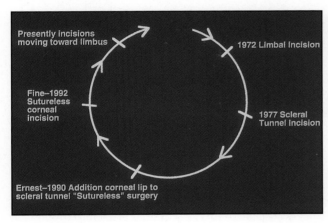

Figure 3-41. Diagram showing the full circle of incisions from 1972 to present.

The phrase "clear corneal incision" still exists, even though the location is more in the anterior limbal area. It is important that surgeons not be confused by this misnomer. The results of all the cadaver work, the human work of the University of Berlin, and the animal work of Dr. Figueiredo, Dr. Tipperman, Dr. Kardassis, and myself all clearly show the advantage of starting in a vascular origin. Dr. Ralph Eagle has demonstrated the histologic response in starting in this area.

Materials

Creation of the Limbal Incision

Following preparation of the patient, a Pierce (Storz, Clearwater, Fla) lid speculum is inserted in the eye. The temporal approach is made. A paracentesis incision is made approximately 20 to 30 degrees away from the proposed cataract incision site. Intracameral lido-

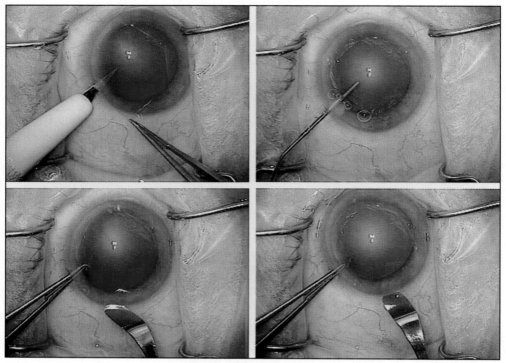

Figure 3-42. A vertical incision in the limbal area.

caine 1.0% (0.2 to 0.3 ml) is instilled in the anterior chamber. A waiting period of 10 seconds is taken. Viscoat (Alcon, Fort Worth, Tex) is instilled in the anterior chamber. 0.12 forceps are inserted through the paracentesis incision, a crescent blade (Alcon) is used to make a vertical incision in the limbal area (Figure 3-42). Dissection is made into the cornea of 2.0 mm (Figure 3-43). A keratome blade of 3.0 mm is then passed up the tunnel and additional incision dissection is carried a little more anteriorly—approximately 0.2 to 0.5 mm—before entering the anterior chamber. This entry into the anterior chamber is accomplished by using the left hand holding the 0.12 forceps and pulling the globe into the tip of the keratome blade. Once Descemet's membrane is broken, the left hand remains still and the right hand holding the keratome blade then passes the blade into the anterior chamber very slowly, creating a linear cut through Descemet's membrane. The left hand helps retract the globe away from the keratome blade as the right hand removes it from the eye. Special care is taken not to make an inadvertent cut at the lateral edges of the tunnel incision, which can extend more anteriorly during manipulation of the wound through phacoemulsification, thereby resulting in an inadequate seal (Figure 3-44).

It is important to note that the amount of viscoelastic instilled in the anterior chamber and the pressure of the eye play a role in the quality of the cut through Descemet's membrane. If the eye is left too soft, it is very easy to have an extra long cut in the corneal tissue, resulting in too anterior an incision and making it longer than it is wide, resulting in oarlocking, corneal edema, and possible encroachment on the visual axis. Too soft an eye may also result in an inadvertent cut to the lateral aspect of the incision externally.

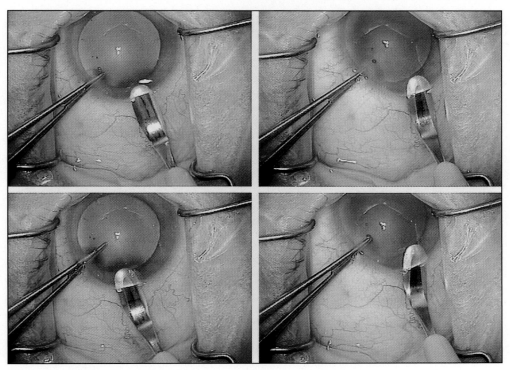

Figure 3-43. Dissection into the cornea.

If the eye is too firm from too much viscoelastic, then entry into the anterior chamber through Descemet's membrane will result in a triangular cut in the same configuration of that of the keratome itself. While this does not necessarily give poor wound closure, it can cause the internal lip to roll in on itself at the end of the procedure, making wound stability less than desirable.

Safe Phacoemulsification

With the use of small incisions, foldable lenses, and topical and intracameral anesthesia, it is important that our phacoemulsification technique be reproducible with minimal complications. Over the past 6 years, I have evaluated my phacoemulsification technique and have standardized the technique to reduce posterior capsular ruptures with or without vitreous loss to an incidence of 1 in 500 worst case scenario to 1 in 1000 best case scenario. I have broken the technique down into four critical areas that must be performed in a mechanical, robot-like fashion in order to achieve these desired results.

The four key areas include:
1. Capsulorrhexis
2. Hydrocortical cleavage and delineating
3. Nuclear disassembly
4. Removal of subincisional cortex

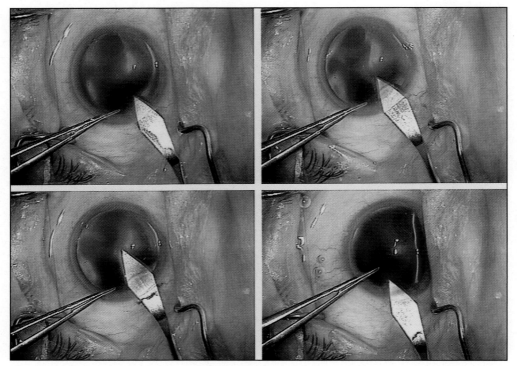

Figure 3-44. Inadvertent cut at the lateral edges of the tunnel incision resulting in an inadequate seal.

Capsulorrhexis

The important part of capsulorrhexis has to do with a reproducible tear of the anterior capsule. Most surgeons will tear the anterior capsule until they find they are running into difficulty and then release the anterior capsule, regrasp it, and continue their tear. I found that if you start in the center of the anterior capsule, creating a small triangular flap to tear either clockwise or counterclockwise, which ever the surgeon prefers. The key to successful capsulorrhexis is to give the same length of tear each and every time and to place the capsule the same length each and every time, one creates muscle memory that allows one to deal with more difficult situations such as white, mature cataracts or a deep, dark, brunescent cataracts in which visualization of the anterior capsule is limited. By placing the capsule centrally before releasing it, viscoelastic is prevented from extruding the anterior capsule through the internal corneal lip, causing an inadvertent extension of the tear of the anterior capsule peripherally. Placing the capsule centrally before releasing it also allows one to regrasp the capsule more easily (Figure 3-45). The desired amount of capsulorrhexis is about 5 to 5.5 mm, depending on the size of the optic of the implant to be used. Under special circumstances where one has a young patient and the anterior chamber is more elastic, one purposely strives for a smaller capsulorrhexis.

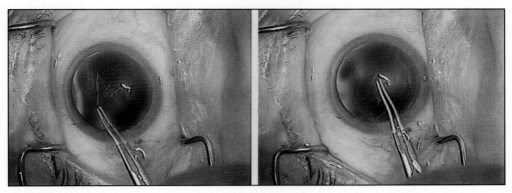

Figure 3-45. Left: capsulorrhexis performed in counter-clockwise fashion. Right: torn capsule is placed centrally before releasing and regrasping.

Hydrocortical Cleavage and Hydrodelineation

Successful hydrocortical cleavage is accomplished using a spatula-type cannula (Visitec, Sarasota, Fla). All air is removed from the cannula before insertion into the eye. The cannula is placed under the end of the anterior capsule and extended peripherally (Figure 3-46). A sideways motion is also used to make sure you are above the anterior-most level of the cortex up against the internal aspect of the anterior capsule. After you are in a proper location, apply pressure to the syringe to inject fluid. The fluid injected should result in a "delayed fluid wave" (see Figure 3-46), an indication that you are in the proper plane. If the fluid wave comes quickly, it is a sign that you are not in the proper plane due to improper placement of the cannula or premature injection of fluid.

Disassembly of the Nucleus

The technique I use in disassembly of the nucleus is as follows: I create perpendicular grooves. I sculpt to a level of approximately 60%, which is 1 to 1.5 phaco tip thicknesses. Since 1991, I have used a 45-degree phaco tip to do the sculpting and a 15-degree phaco tip to remove the nuclear quadrant. With newer technology, the 30-degree micro tip by Kellman can be used throughout. The sculpting process is not only at a depth of 60%, which gives a margin of safety, but it also does not extent very peripherally. Sculpting only goes up to the edge of the capsulorrhexis. This safety prevents any damage to the anterior capsule, which can result in inadvertent anterior capsular tear that can extend posteriorly, resulting in complications of vitreous loss or dropped nucleus.

After I have completed the perpendicular grooves, I inject Viscoat into the anterior chamber. I use the Ernest nuclear cracker (Katina, Denville, NJ) to crack the nucleus into four quadrants. The Ernest nuclear cracker allows the forceps to be used through a wound size of 2.5 mm. It gives wide extension of the paddles for adequate cracking. The wide surface area of the paddles gives adequate force to crack the nucleus with grooves 60% in depth. It has a tapered posterior aspect for easy removal over the internal corneal ledge. By cracking under viscoelastic, one has total control. One can rotate the nucleus and ensure that the quadrants are adequately separated from one another before proceeding to nucleus removal (Figures 3-47a and 3-47b).

Each quadrant is then engaged and emulsified (Figure 3-48). The epinucleus is left

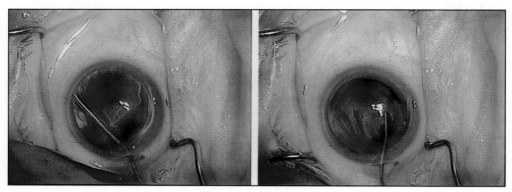

Figure 3-46. Cannula placed under the end of the anterior capsule and extended peripherally.

behind to give adequate protection to the posterior capsule. An additional amount of viscoelastic may be injected if there is compromised corneal endothelium or if it is necessary to position the remaining quadrant for easy access.

Pulse-mode phaco can be used in removing the last quadrant to reduce chatter of the nuclear fragment. Pulse-mode phaco can be used with aspiration to remove the epinucleus and cortical material.

Phaco Chop

Phaco chop, as described by Dr. Kunihiro Nagahara of Japan, can also be used with this technique. After disassembly of the nucleus into four quadrants, a chopping instrument can be used to help break off smaller pieces of the quadrant if these quadrants are excessively large due to asymmetrical cracking or if they are extremely dense. It is easier to chop a quadrant than it is to chop an entire nucleus in half, or half a nucleus into smaller quadrants. It is less risky to the anterior capsulorrhexis in chopping quadrants and less likely to cause an anterior capsular slip, which can result in a posterior capsular tear.

Removal of Subincisional Cortex

It is imperative that subincisional cortex be removed using a bimanual irrigation-aspiration technique. If one uses a conventional irrigation-aspiration handpiece, subincisional cortex should be removed only after an intraocular lens is properly placed. With posterior chamber intraocular lens in the capsular bag, one can use a right-angle irrigation-aspiration tip to engage and remove all subincisional cortex. The aspiration tip is blunt and the aspiration port is on the internal side. The tip is used to push the implant posteriorly, creating a cleft. The aspiration port can easily engage the cortical material for removal (Figure 3-49). It is important to note that the haptics of a multipiece lens, or the foot plate in a single-piece lens, must be directed away from the subincisional cortex so that trapping of cortical material at the equator of the capsule is prevented.

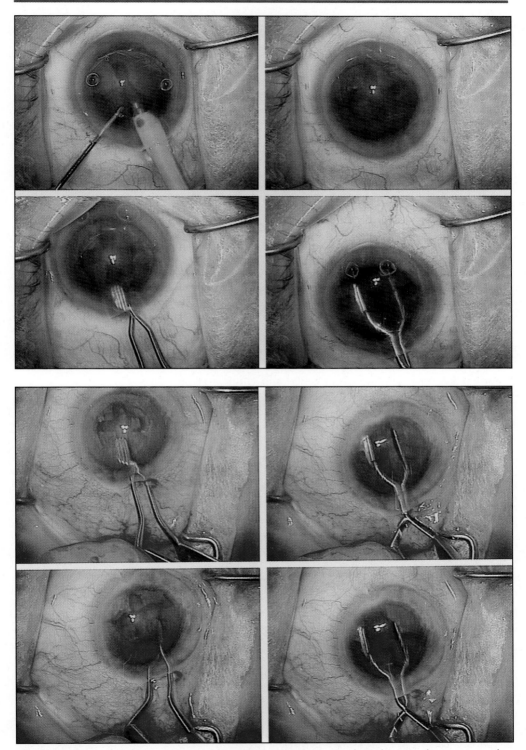

Figures 3-47a and b. Rotation of the nuclear to ensure that the quadrants are adequately separated from one another before proceeding to nuclear removal.

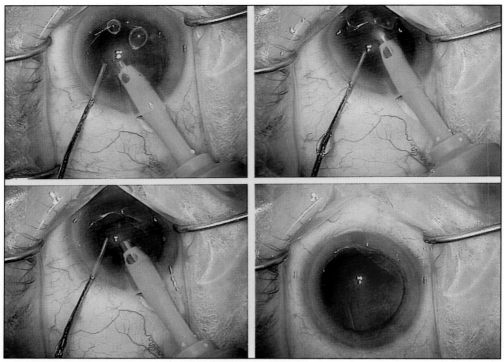

Figure 3-48. Each quadrant is engaged and emulsified.

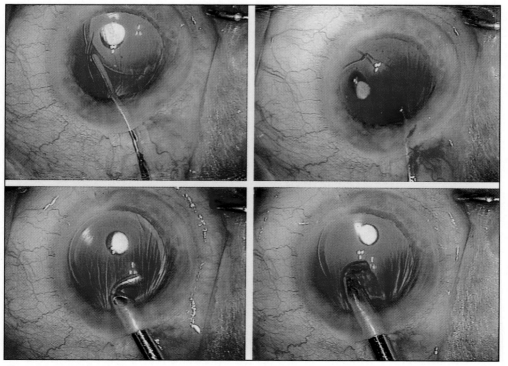

Figure 3-49. The aspiration port can easily engage the cortical material for removal.

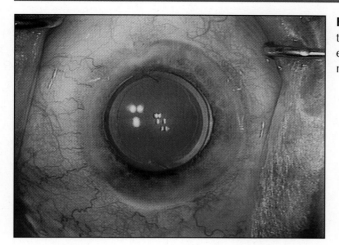

Figure 3-50. BSS is instilled in the anterior chamber to ensure that the internal lip is not rolled inward on itself.

Testing of the Incision

Upon the completion of the technique, balanced salt solution is instilled in the anterior chamber to ensure that the internal lip is not rolled inward on itself (Figure 3-50). The wound is tested on high and low pressure to ensure that the wound is stable. With a relatively square incision that is 3 mm in width and 2.5. to 3 mm in length it is not necessary to use stromal hydration. Throughout the entire procedure, antibiotics are used in the balanced salt solution, including all the syringes filled with balanced salt solution. The composition of the antibiotics is as follows: 500 cc balanced salt solution, 20 mg Vancomycin (Lilly, Indianapolis, Ind), and 10 mg Tobramycin (Lilly).

Foreign Body Sensation

It has been noted by colleagues that foreign body sensation is a real problem in patients with a corneal incision with a vertical component. The reason for this is as one performs surgery through a corneal incision with a vertical component, one creates edema on both the anterior and posterior aspects of the incision (Figures 3-51 and 3-52). This creates a trough foreign body sensation that can last up to 1 year post-surgery (Figure 3-53). If one uses the limbal site (Figures 3-54 and 3-55). The only edema is in the tunnel of the incision and foreign body sensation is remarkably reduced (Figure 3-56).

Conclusion

Intraocular lens technology and phacoemulsification technology has allowed surgeons to tremendously reduce the size of their incisions. Most surgeries can now be performed through incisions of approximately 3 mm in width. Using a limbal incision, one can have all of the advantages of aesthetics and efficiency of surgery, still have the stability of a relatively square incision, the ability to stretch the tissue due to elastic fibers and have it return to its normal configuration, have a reduction in foreign body sensation, and a fast healing process through a fibroblastic response.

Figure 3-51. Schematic demonstrating the clear corneal incision with a vertical component.

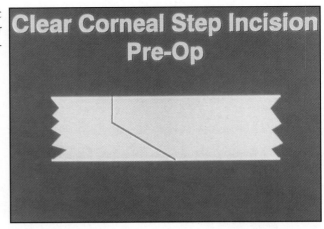

Figure 3-52. Schematic demonstrating the clear corneal incision with a vertical component.

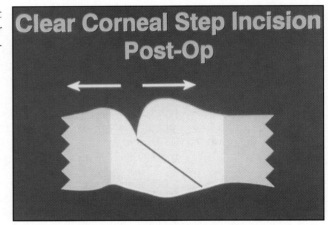

Figure 3-53. One-day postoperative result on a patient with a clear corneal incision showing foreign body sensation.

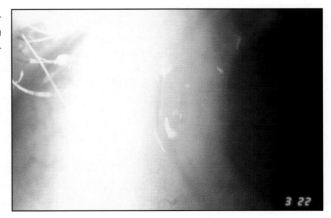

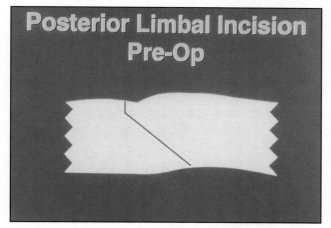

Figure 3-54. Schematic representation of a limbal incision.

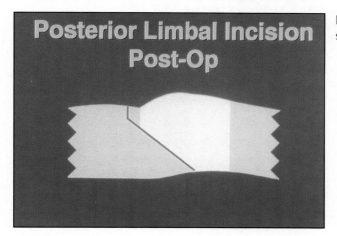

Figure 3-55. Schematic representation of a limbal incision.

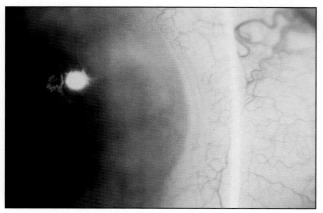

Figure 3-56. One-day postoperative limbal incision with no foreign body sensation.

References

1. Ernest PH, Kiessling LA, Lavery KT. Relative strength of cataract incisions in cadaver eyes. *J Cataract Refract Surg.* 1991;17(Suppl):668-671.

2. Koch PS. Structural analysis of cataract incision construction. *J Cataract Refract Surg.* 1991;17(Suppl):661-667.

3. Obstbaum SA. Wound construction and closure: steps for improved stability in cataract surgery (editorial). *J Cataract Refract Surg.* 1991;17(Suppl):659.

4. Ernest PH. Wound stability. *J Cataract Refract Surg.* 1989;Jan.

5. Ernest PH, Kiessling LA, Lavery KT. Relative strength of cataract incisions in cadaver eyes. *J Cataract Refract Surg.* 1991;17(Suppl):668-671.

6. Ernest PH, Lavery KT, Kiessling LA. Relative strength of scleral tunnel incisions with internal corneal lips constructed in cadaver eyes. *J Cataract Refract Surg.* 1993;19:457-461.

7. Masket S. One year postoperative astigmatic comparison of sutured and unsutured 4.0 mm scleral pocket incisions. *J Cataract Refract Surg.* 1993;19:453-456.

8. DeFigueiredo CG. Relative strength of clear corneal incision sealed by organic glue in the rabbit eye. Presented at the American Society of Cataract and Refractive Surgery annual meeting. April 1995, San Diego, Calif.

9. Ernest PH, Tipperman R, Kardassis C, Lavery KT, Sensoli AM. The healing process based on incision location. Presented at the American Society of Cataract and Refractive Surgery annual meeting. June 1996, Seattle, Wash.

4

Endophthalmitis: Scleral Tunnel vs. Clear Corneal Incision

Maurice E. John, MD
Randall Noblitt, OD

This chapter is included in this book to highlight the potential problems with endophthalmitis with the clear corneal incision. While the study compares scleral tunnel to clear corneal surgery, the blue line incision is essentially equivalent to the scleral tunnel incision in this regard. We feel this chapter clearly shows the increased risk of clear corneal lens-based surgery.

Introduction

Clear corneal cataract incisions, first described by Fine as "self-sealing corneal tunnel incision for small-incision cataract surgery," (*Ocular Surgery News*, May 1, 1992), involved a straight-in entry beginning at the edge of clear cornea. The stability of this incision seemed to be due to its temporal location.[1] Its simplicity and ease of construction has made the technique popular, with no published reports of complications.

However, anecdotal reports of an increased incidence in endophthalmitis has, over time, led to proposed changes to the procedure to increase the security of the closure. Very shortly after we began performing the procedure, we started making a two-plane incision by first making a perpendicular groove before incising with a keratome 1.5 to 2 mm into the cornea. We consistently checked for leaks immediately after surgery and, for reduced intraocular pressures, 1 day after surgery, and this incision always appeared watertight.

However, a perceived increase in sterile endophthalmitis over the next 4 years led to this retrospective study. We collected all primary cataract surgeries performed during this period to determine the relative incidence of sterile endophthalmitis in clear corneal incisions using our two-plane architecture compared with the incidence among scleral-tunnel incisions using a three-plane architecture during the same period of time.

Methods

Surgical Techniques

All procedures were performed by two surgeons at John-Kenyon Eye Center using identical incision techniques. The clear corneal technique was performed as follows: sodium brevital followed by a periocular block using 5 cc of 2% Xylocaine (Abbott Labs, Chicago, Ill) with epinephrine and Wydase were administered. A super pinky was placed on the eye. After approximately 30 minutes, the patient was taken to the operating room and placed under monitored anesthesia care, prepped, and draped in the usual manner. The eyelids were taped open and flooded with Ocuflox (Allergan, Irvine, Calif).

A John groover knife (Mastel) set at 0.26 mm depth was used to create a 2.7 to 3.2 mm perpendicular groove at the clear cornea, temporally. A paracentesis was created 3 clock hours to the right. A diamond keratome was used to enter the anterior chamber. The resulting incision was 1.5 to 2 mm in length and 2.8 to 3.2 mm in width. Viscoelastic was instilled. A 360-degree tear capsulorrhexis was performed, followed by hydrodissection. Phacoemulsification, irrigation, and aspiration of all cortical remnants was performed. The 500 ml balanced saline irrigating solution contained 0.1 ml Garamycin (APP, Los Angeles, Calif), 0.2 ml Vancomycin, 800 microns of heparin, and 0.5 ml adrenaline. The irrigating solution was filtered as described by Gills.[2]

The lens was loaded into the injector and placed into the bag. Irrigation and aspiration was then performed. Vancomycin was injected through the sideport to restore pressure. The wound was checked for watertightness visually and left sutureless. A drop each of pilocarpine 4%, Ocuflox, Betoptic (Alcon, Fort Worth, Tex), Voltaren (Alcon), and Pred Forte were instilled. A patch was applied.

The scleral tunnel procedure was performed as follows: the patient was prepared for surgery as described above. A limbal-based flap was lifted and the limbus cauterized. A partial thickness 2.8- to 3.2-mm incision was made. A sideport incision was made 3 clock hours to the right. The 2.8-mm incision was then dissected forward with a spoon blade. The keratome was used to enter the anterior chamber. The procedure was then completed as previously described.

Our prophylactic regimen for all cases was as follows: patients received preoperative and immediate postoperative topical antibiotics. The 500 ml balanced saline irrigating solution was filtered and also contained 0.1 ml Garamycin and 0.2 ml Vancomycin. Vancomycin was injected into the anterior chamber immediately at the conclusion of the case. Patients received a 1-week course of Tobradex, which was then replaced by Pred Forte for 3 to 4 weeks.

Data Collection and Analysis

All primary cataract extractions performed between July 1, 1992 and October 31, 1996 were collected from the charts. Patients receiving combined procedures were excluded. The cases were grouped into two cohorts, which were followed prospectively using the medical charts. The two cohorts were defined by determining whether a two-plane clear corneal or scleral tunnel incision had been performed. The endpoint of interest was the occurrence of endophthalmitis within the first 3 months postoperatively. Endophthalmitis was indicated in the chart if the patient had presented with characteristic signs (ie, hypopyon, pain, photophobia, and/or decreasing vision). All cases that had presented with symptoms of endophthalmitis were cultured and referred to retinal specialists.

The incidence rate of endophthalmitis was determined for each group and compared between groups using a test of binomial proportions. An odds ratio was computed, which is the relative risk (between the two incision groups) of having endophthalmitis.[3]

Results

A total of 8346 procedures were evaluated, of which 3126 were two-plane clear corneal incisions and 5216 were scleral tunnel incisions. Ten cases of sterile endophthalmitis occurred, which is an overall incidence of 0.12%. Nine of those had received a clear corneal incision (incidence = 0.29%), and one a scleral tunnel incision (incidence = 0.02%). These rates were statistically significantly different between the two groups (p<0.006, binomial test of proportions). The odds ratio (relative risk) of developing endophthalmitis for clear corneal procedures versus scleral tunnel procedures was 12.5 (SE = 13.2). All 10 cases of endophthalmitis were culture negative. No cases of culture positive endophthalmitis in primary cataract extraction occurred during this period.

Among the sterile endophthalmitis cases, procedures were performed between October 6, 1992 and October 14, 1996. Seven were performed by one surgeon, and three by the other surgeon. Nuclear density varied between grades 1 and 3.5. Plate-haptic silicone lenses were used in nine cases (three by Chiron and six by STAAR), and one case received an AMO silicon lens. Average surgery time was 7 minutes with a range of 4 to 12.

Patients presented with symptoms from 2 to 36 days postoperatively, with a mean of 13. Mean age was 75.7 years. Seventy percent were female. Mean 1-day intraocular pressure (IOP) was 18.6 mmHg. At the time of diagnosis, three patients had VAsc between 20/50 and 20/80, and seven patients were worse than 20/100. After the infection resolved, four cases could see 20/25 or better and five could see between 20/30 and 20/40. One case with pre-existing macular degeneration had VAsc of 20/50.

Discussion

Langerman[3] and Ernest[4] have shown that both straight-in and two-plane clear corneas can leak. This ability to leak indicates a less than perfect seal, even though the wound may appear watertight and the 1-day pressure is normal. Because of the relatively long period between surgery and symptomalogy in many of our cases, it is unlikely in those cases that infection was caused by unsterile surgical technique. It is more probable that there was a reflux of normal flora into the anterior chamber through the incision.

Reported rates of endophthalmitis in phacoemulsification have ranged from 0.015% to 0.74%.[5,6] Overall incidence of endophthalmitis in our center is well within that range (0.12%); thus, it is unlikely that our endophthalmitis cases would be due to improper procedures or poor surgery.

Our aggressive prophylactic regimen probably accounts for our lack of culture-positive endophthalmitis. In 8342 cases, we did not have a single case of active infection. A recent survey (Samuel Masket, MD, *ASCRS Endophthalmitis Survey*, presented at the American Society of Cataract and Refractive Surgery, 1997) suggests the use of postoperative topical antibiotics and antibiotics in the infusate reduces the risk of culture-positive infection.

Modifications to the clear corneal incisions that may improve watertightness have been proposed. Fine has suggested irrigating balanced salt solution (BSS) into the edges of the incision to hydrate it and increase closure. Langerman[3] has proposed a hinge technique, which involves making the initial vertical groove deeper than the point at which the horizontal shelf is started. The deep groove then functions as a hinge, keeping the wound sealed. Since February 1996, one of the authors (Maurice John, MD) has adopted the hinge technique, making the initial groove at a 0.6 mm depth perpendicular to the cornea and then constructing a 1.75 to 2 mm incision through the superficial cornea. The author presses on the incision with a cellulose sponge for 20 seconds, as proposed by Hoffer (American College of Eye Surgeons, February 1996) to aid in adhesion of the tissues. A second sponge is held over the visual axis to protect the macula.

Between February 1996 and October 1996, 623 hinged incisions as described above were performed with no incidence of endophthalmitis. During the same period with the older technique, two cases occurred. Recently, we have made another modification by moving the incision temporally about 0.33 mm to include the capillaries. Although surgical technique has moved toward limiting or eliminating hyphema, blood may actually increase the rapidity of healing and closure of the incision.

Just as the scleral tunnel incision underwent changes and development from its original description by Dr. Masket[7] to a sutureless, superficial tunnel incision,[8] the clear corneal incision can be made safer by new developments. We believe that based on our comparative rates of endophthalmitis, the clear corneal incision, as originally described, should be abandoned. Surgeons should make one or more of the proposed modifications to their clear corneal incision technique to ensure a more complete closure. Of course, the scleral tunnel sutureless wound remains an excellent alternative.

References

1. Fine IH, Fichman RA, Grabow HB, eds. *Clear-Corneal Cataract Surgery and Topical Anesthesia.* Thorofare, NJ: SLACK Incorporated; 1993.

2. Gills JP. Prevention of endophthalmitis by intraocular solution filtration and antibiotics. *American Intra-Ocular Implant Society Journal.* 1985;11:185-186.

3. Langerman DW. Architectural design of a self-sealing corneal tunnel, single-hinge incision. *J Cataract Refract Surg.* 1994;20:84-88.

4. Ernest PH, Fenzl R, Lavery KT, Sensoli A. Relative stability of clear corneal incisions in a cadaver eye model. *J Cataract Refract Surg.* 1995;21:39-42.

5. Williams DL, Gills JP. Infectious endophthalmitis following sutureless cataract surgery (letter). *Arch Ophthalmol.* 1992;110:913.

6. Powe NR, Schein O, Geiser S, et al. Synthesis of the literature on visual acuity and complications following cataract extraction with intraocular lens implantation. *Arch Ophthalmol.* 1994;112:239-252.

7. Masket S. Astigmatic analysis of the scleral pocket incision and closure technique for cataract surgery. *CLAO Journal.* 1985;11:206-209.

8. John M, Noblitt R, Boleyn K, et al. The effect of a superficial and a deep scleral pocket on the incidence of hyphema. *J Cataract Refract Surg.* 1992;18:495-499.

The Blue Line Cataract Incision

5

Jean-Luc Febbraro, MD
Kurt A. Buzard, MD, FACS

Historical Introduction

The cataract incision is a subject that has received intense scrutiny over the past several years but is a subject of perineal interest and, in a sense, has defined the state of cataract surgery at any given time.[1,2,3,4,5] George Waring has stated that "the introduction of the Graefe's incision for the cataract surgery introduced not only the birth of modern cataract surgery, but also a century-long epidemic of surgically induced corneal astigmatism" due to the propensity of this sutureless corneal incision to induce large amounts of astigmatism.[6] Shiotz described a 33-year-old patient who developed 19.5 diopters (D) of astigmatism after a Graefe's cataract incision (Figure 5-1), which he treated with an *ab interno* incision reducing the astigmatism to 7 D![7] The intimate association between induced astigmatism and cataract incision continues to this day and will be one of the subjects discussed in this chapter in the comparison between the clear corneal and blue line incision.

The method of entrance into the eye is one of the most frequent causes of complications, and subsequent visual improvement is heavily dependent on the success (or failure) of the cataract incision. The beginning of the modern cataract incision era was marked by the onset of sutureless incisions. McFarland introduced sutureless cataract surgery in January 1990 after observing that scleral tunnel incisions were watertight without sutures when the wound was properly constructed (Figures 5-2 and 5-3).[5] As the size of the incision has been reduced, the location of the external entry has shifted from the more traditional scleral tunnel toward the clear corneal approach. In 1992, Fine observed self-sealing clear corneal tunnel incisions and additionally found that such incisions could be placed in a temporal location (Figures 5-4 to 5-6).[3]

The reasons for this shift in technique have been many, but increased efficiency, reduced requirement for cautery (thus reducing postoperative astigmatism), and the trend toward topical anesthesia have been significant reasons. Today, the clear corneal incision has been adopted by an increasing number of surgeons; however, it necessitates nearly perfect wound architecture to obtain a watertight closure. In addition, within the ring of the limbus, incisions inevitably create astigmatism, and this incision is no different. While the incision is supposed to be a benefit when performed on the steep axis, the correction is variable and

Figure 5-1. Graeffe cataract incision showing the steps of the standard incision.

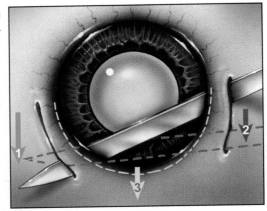

Figure 5-2. Top view of a scleral tunnel incision showing a roughly square incision with good self-sealing characteristics.

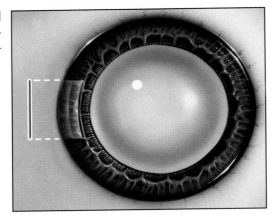

Figure 5-3. Side view of a stepped scleral tunnel incision.

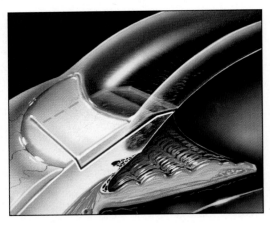

irregular, and in the best of circumstances, only an acceptable compromise. In the problem cases, irregular astigmatism can lead to a loss of best-corrected vision. The clear corneal incision is not forgiving and can lead to several undesirable complications, such as wound leakage, postoperative endophthalmitis, and irregular astigmatism, especially for inexperienced surgeons.

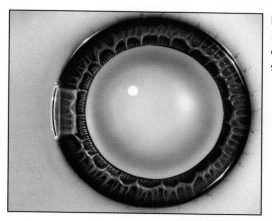

Figure 5-4. Top view of a clear corneal incision showing rectangular incision configuration with slightly poorer self-sealing characteristics.

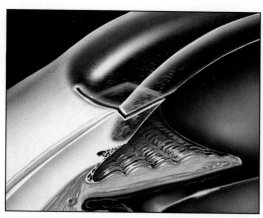

Figure 5-5. Side view of a stepped clear corneal incision.

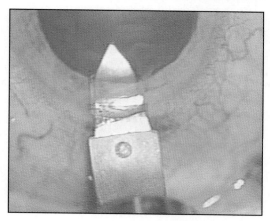

Figure 5-6. Clinical view of a clear corneal incision showing avascular entry and rectangular incision configuration.

Ernest and Neuhann have promoted the concept of moving the external entrance of the incision more posteriorly into the bloody edge of the limbus so as to promote better wound healing (Figure 5-7).[8,9] While the benefits of this relatively small posterior movement are clear, we believe that even greater benefits (more predictable wound closure, more flexibility for extension and suturing, and more convenience in terms of grasping the lip of the

Figure 5-7. Top view of bloody limbal incision showing fixation with instrument in side port.

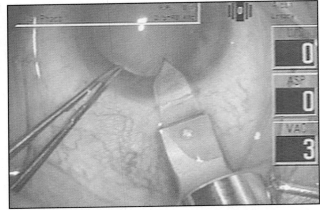

Figure 5-8. Limbal anatomy showing bluish area between sclera and cornea.

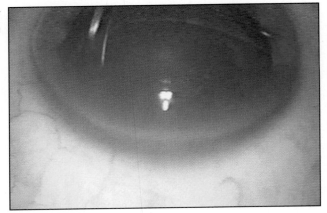

wound) can be obtained by placing the incision even further posteriorly—1 to 2 mm from the surgical limbus at a location seen through the conjunctiva to be a bluish line (Figures 5-8 and 5-9). While it might seem that a peritomy is necessary in this location, we have found that a diamond incision through the conjunctiva at the blue line can create a "mini-peritomy" that does not develop chemosis during an efficient phacoemulsification. The blue line that we use in this context is not the blue line that has been discussed in the past at the limbus. In this context, the blue line is posterior to the limit of the firm adherence of the conjunctiva to the sclera, approximately 2 mm from the surgical limbus. At this location, the conjunctiva ends firm adherence to the sclera and becomes mobile. The external landmarks of the surgical limbus include a bluish translucent zone, 1 to 1.2 mm wide at the superior limbus, when the conjunctiva is removed. This bluish translucent zone is located posteriorly to the anterior limbal border and is visible if the limbus is dissected free of conjunctiva. With the conjunctiva intact, the anatomical landmarks change and the bluish area now visible between the cornea and sclera represents an area approximately 2 mm wide, in which the conjunctiva is firmly attached to the sclera. We have defined the blue line as the posterior aspect of this zone and we place the incision in this location (Figures 5-10 and 5-11) because with the firm attachment anterior to the incision, no chemosis forms and posterior to the incision, a natural mini-peritomy forms with sagging of the mobile conjunctiva.

The initial reaction of an incision through the conjunctiva would be that of concern

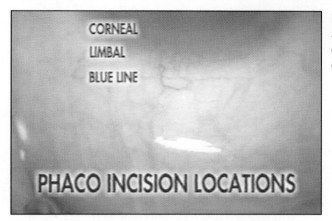

Figure 5-9. Labeled corneal anatomy showing locations of corneal, limbal, and blue line cataract incision.

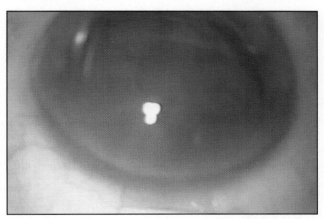

Figure 5-10. First step of the transconjunctival blue line incision showing an incision through conjunctiva using the side of the diamond knife approximately 4 mm in length.

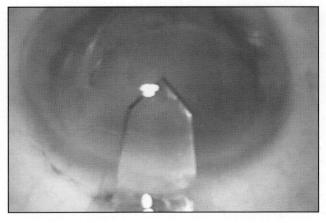

Figure 5-11. Top view clinical photo of diamond insertion in a blue line incision with 3 mm external opening and 2.5 mm width at the "shoulders" of the diamond.

about chemosis during the surgical procedure. In fact, as we will discuss in the Technique section, the initial pass of the diamond knife creates an instant mini-peritomy that does not become chemotic with an efficient phacoemulsification. Therefore, part of the successful implementation of the blue line incision is efficiency in the removal and replacement of the lens, which we will consider in Chapter 6. In summary, we believe that the blue line inci-

Figure 5-12. Artist's rendition of the first step of the blue line incision showing cutting of conjunctiva with the diamond knife 4 mm in length.

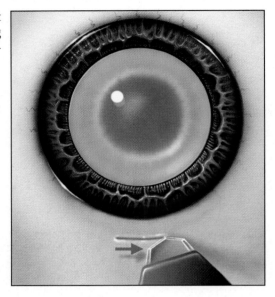

sion retains many of the benefits of the clear corneal incision, combining its efficiency with the safety and benefits of the more traditional scleral tunnel incision. As such, we see this incision as the endpoint for several groups of surgeons. For those surgeons currently using a scleral tunnel approach, a simple transition allows greater efficiency with the same approach. For the clear corneal surgeons looking for greater wound strength, better wound healing, and more convenient surgery, the blue line incision is also a natural choice.

Surgical Technique

In general terms, the blue line incision is more convenient to perform than a comparable clear corneal incision because of the ability to grasp the wound edge for stabilization when inserting instruments. In outline form, the incision is created by one pass of the side of the diamond knife to create the mini-peritomy (Figure 5-12), a second single stab to enter the eye (Figure 5-13), and a light cautery is used to control minor bleeding (Figure 5-14). During the incision construction, the eye is exposed, drawn downward, and stabilized by grasping in the inferior conjunctiva with a .5 forceps. We believe that this fixation technique for the initial incision is as effective yet simpler than other techniques, such as holding the eye with a ring or with an instrument inserted into the side port.

The blue line incision is constructed by first creating a 4-mm incision through the conjunctiva with the side of the diamond knife about 1.5 to 2 mm behind the surgical limbus (represented by an anatomic appearance of a blue line). In the usual case, the conjunctiva naturally sags away from the incision and the resulting conjunctival gaping creates a mini-peritomy (Figure 5-15a). While bleeding is not a significant problem, the assistant applies steady drops to maintain visualization of the exterior incision, and light cautery is applied when the incision is completed.

The knife is placed parallel to the posterior sclera and pressure is applied to slightly indent the sclera with the knife, pushing forward to begin the scleral tunnel incision (Figure

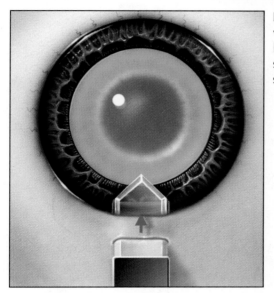

Figure 5-13. Artist's rendition of top view of diamond insertion in the blue line incision showing approximately square incision configuration and straight interior tunnel opening.

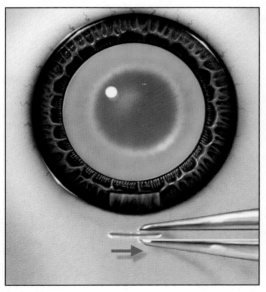

Figure 5-14. Artist's rendition of light cautery applied after the incision.

5-15b). A scleral groove is not performed, but the tip of the knife is used to trace the external incision and cut any remaining tenon's tissue (see Figures 5-10 and 5-12). During the scleral tunnel construction, progressive pressure is applied on the heel of the diamond knife to prevent early interior entry caused by the changing curvature at the limbus between the sclera and cornea (Figure 5-15c). Finally, when the tip of the knife has approached the desired location for the internal corneal incision, the heel of the knife is rotated slightly upward and the pressure is transferred toward the tip of the knife. At that point, a slight dimple is visible in the corneal surface that disappears when the knife penetrates into the anterior chamber (Figure 5-15d). The knife is then inserted until the "shoulders" are at the level of the internal corneal incision, which is 2.5 mm in width (see Figure 5-11). The blue

Figure 5-15. A: Schematic illustration of mini-peritomy after transconjunctival incision 2 mm from the limbus. **B:** Schematic illustration of knife insertion beginning with downward applanation of the diamond with forward movement. **C:** Schematic illustration of diamond insertion showing the tip of the diamond at the limbus, at which point the heel of the diamond is rotated downward to keep the tip of diamond within the cornea. **D:** Schematic illustration of the final step of diamond insertion in which the location for the anterior extent of the cataract incision is identified, the heel of the diamond is rotated upward, creating a "dimple" in the cornea with subsequent entrance of the diamond into the anterior chamber.

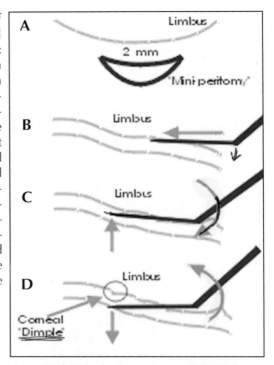

Figure 5-16. Side view of blue line transconjunctival incision showing an identical profile as a scleral tunnel incision.

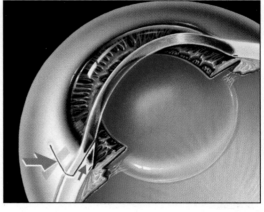

line incision described above results in an approximately square 3 x 3 mm transconjunctival corneoscleral incision (Figure 5-16). Light cautery is then applied to the conjunctival edge to control bleeding (see Figure 5-14). We use the same knife to create the side incision port through the bloody edge of the posterior limbus. This creates a very desirable incision configuration with a wide exterior incision and a narrow interior port. Manipulation through the side port causes little corneal distortion and the incision closes easily.

At the end of the cataract procedure, wound integrity is checked with the wound leakage test, which is performed by injecting saline through the side port, checking along the incision by drying with a sponge, and applying some pressure on the sclera (Figure 5-17). Of interest is the fact that hydration of the cornea, frequently required to obtain a watertight

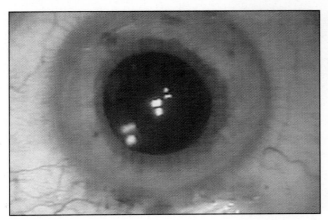

Figure 5-17. Clinical photo of a blue line incision at the conclusion of the case showing watertight closure and positioning of the incision.

wound in the clear corneal incision, is rarely required with the blue line incision. While sutureless wound closure is rarely a problem with this incision, a few comments on this topic are appropriate. One reason closure of a small incision might be impeded would be stretching of the scleral and corneal fibers near the incision. The longer the operation lasts and the more phacoemulsification energy is used, the more stretched these fibers become—a good argument for an efficient surgery. As a personal observation, corneal fibers are more prone to stretching than scleral tissue, and the scleral tunnel of the blue line incision is therefore slightly more resistant to stretching than a comparable clear corneal incision. One useful maneuver is hydration of the cornea, which takes up the slack in the corneal fibers and closes the wound. Another useful maneuver is elevating intraocular pressure in a relatively rapid manner, allowing the wound to reorient itself and close. Finally, moderate cautery at the ends of the incision can induce a small amount of scleral contraction and help seal the external mouth of the incision, acting almost like a horizontal suture. In our relatively extensive experience with the blue line incision (several thousand cases), we have never seen a wound leak through the primary cataract incision.

One final point concerns the use of cautery. We use cautery sparingly in the beginning of the surgery and most bleeding has resolved by the end of surgery. In most cases, very light bleeding is resolved by additional cautery, applied primarily at the ends of the incisions at the end of the case. In our experience, induced astigmatism from cautery is not a feature of this incision, and 1-day uncorrected vision reflects this fact, as we will discuss later in this chapter.

Instrumentation

The selection of the appropriate knife to perform a cataract incision needs to be carefully considered, as the construction of the incision depends on the type of blade—its length, width, and thickness. We create the incision with a trapezoid diamond knife that has a 2.5 mm inside diameter and a 3.0 mm outside width. This knife is longer (8 mm) than the standard cataract diamond knife, allowing for the more posterior placement of the external wound. In addition, the tip of the knife is truncated (100 microns) to allow for better control in tissue and placement of the internal corneal wound (Figures 5-18 and 5-19). This knife's properties provide the ideal sharpness and precision during the wound construction.

Figure 5-18. Photograph of Mastel Stealth diamond knife showing a truncated tip and trapezoidal configuration (Mastel Precision, Rapid City, SD).

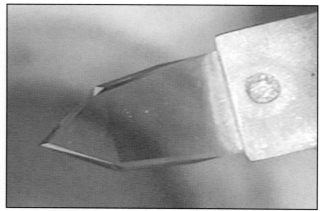

Figure 5-19. Photograph of Mastel Stealth diamond knife showing the side view and top facet configuration (Mastel Precision, Rapid City, SD).

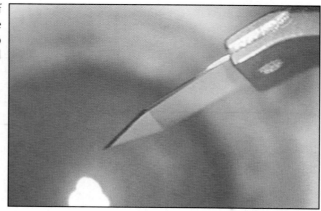

We feel a diamond blade is the best option in cataract surgery in terms of sharpness and durability. Metal knives, even of hardened steel, cannot reach the level of sharpness obtained with a diamond knife. Thus, they create ragged incisions, particularly on the internal incision, which can lead to stripping of Descemet and difficulty in maintaining a watertight closure. In addition, they require higher pressure during the wound construction with possible wound distortion as the globe is fixated with a ring or an instrument is inserted through the side port (Figure 5-20).

The optimal diamond knife should have the length to perform the longer scleral tunnel incision and facets that encourage a good initial incision depth while not promoting premature entry in the anterior chamber. This trapezoid diamond knife has been specifically developed with Mastel Precision (Rapid City, SD) for a scleral tunnel cataract incision. It has a 30 angulated dop and its length (8 mm) is slightly superior to a standard clear corneal incision knife in order to allow for a more posterior wound approach and a longer tunnel. The tip of the blade, which is 100 microns thick, is used to trace the external incision and cut remaining adherent tenon tissues. The trapezoid shape of the blade allows for an almost square scleral tunnel architecture (see Figure 5-16). The pointed part of the blade is 2.5 mm wide and 1.35 mm long and has a truncated tip that enables the knife to float into the tissue during the tunnel construction. The width of the blade progressively increases up to 3.0 mm at its shoulders (see Figure 5-18). The leading edge of the blade has asymmetric facets

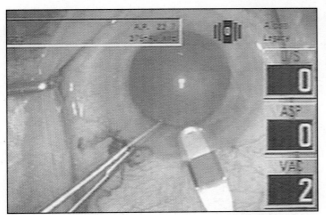

Figure 5-20. Photo of fixation technique in a clear corneal incision through the side port using a metal knife showing torsion on the cornea.

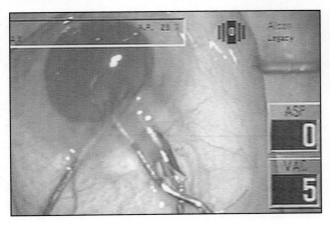

Figure 5-21. Photo of fixation technique in a clear corneal incision through theside port with insertion of an IOL showing torsion on the cornea.

like a spatulated needle, which helps to avoid a premature entrance into the anterior chamber and reduces the need to dimple down when entry into the anterior chamber is performed. This knife was specifically developed to perform the blue line incision and therefore enables a reliable and precise construction of this square (3 x 3 mm) incision.

Advantages and Disadvantages

The blue line incision has many advantages, which have been discussed earlier. In general, the incision allows a rapid and safe entrance into the eye and, in addition, allows the surgery itself to proceed with more facility. When a clear corneal incision is employed, the stabilization of the globe is a significant issue. If a ring fixation is employed, the globe is imperfectly secured, even with teeth on the ring. In fact, the teeth can make fixation even more difficult since they may hurt the patient. In addition, once the knife enters the eye, the increase in intraocular pressure may cause an untimely collapse of the anterior chamber if the entry gapes the wound. A way to avoid this problem is to make the stab incision and then fill the chamber with viscoelastic, although viscoelastic may be wasted if the wound gapes. Another fixation technique involves the use of a second instrument placed through the stab incision (Figures 5-20 and 5-21). This technique is inherently problematic since the

Figure 5-22. Photo of fixation technique in a blue line incision showing the ability to grasp the scleral edge when inserting the phacoemulsification tip.

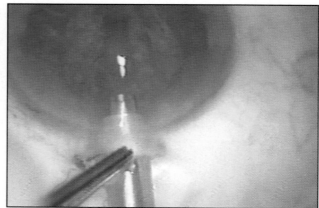

Figure 5-23. Photo of fixation technique in the blue line incision showing the ability to grasp the scleral edge when inserted.

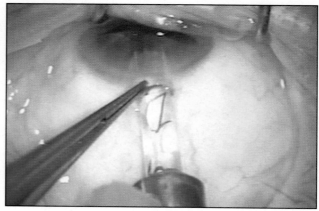

forces applied to the globe are at right angles to the fixation. As a result, the stab incision is gaped open and distorted, resulting in a loss of chamber if viscoelastic is not inserted prior to the procedure. In addition, endothelial cells may be lost and the stab incision my be difficult to close at the conclusion of the case. A better method is to grasp the conjunctiva and tenons 180 degrees away from the incision with a 0.5 forceps and to use this method to both rotate the globe and expose the incision site and to rotate the globe toward the surgeon in a "two-handed" technique as the incision is created. This allows a great deal of accuracy in the placement of the interior aspect of the incision, unlike the two methods previously described in which the stability of the eye is uneven and the entrance is more haphazard. In addition, the wound does not gape with the symmetrical and balanced forces on the eye and wound, meaning no viscoelastic needs be instilled prior to the creation of the incision.

One very significant advantage of the blue line incision is the ability to further stabilize the globe by means of grasping the wound margin as the phacoemulsification tip, I/A tip, and lens are inserted into the eye (Figures 5-22 and 5-23). In addition, entry into the eye does not elevate intraocular pressure or torque the globe, enhancing the stability of the anterior chamber. This is, of course, not practical with the clear corneal incision since the fragile tissue may well be torn away, resulting in a very difficult closure. In fact, the corneal incision itself is an unforgiving incision, particularly if one avoids the groove (which Dr. Fine believes contributes to induced astigmatism, personal communication). Any miscoordina-

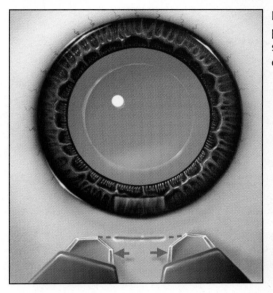

Figure 5-24. Artist's rendition of the simplicity of extending the blue line incision to allow for insertion of a larger IOL or removal of lens material.

tion may cut the sides of the corneal tunnel, or if the knife is directed downward too quickly, the resulting incision may not be watertight. In contrast, the blue line incision pierces through a portion of the sclera before entering the cornea, providing a margin of safety during which the knife may find the proper position. This means the incision may be placed in the most convenient location for the surgeon, either superiorly or temporally if so desired. This aspect of the incision will ease the transition for surgeons currently performing the scleral tunnel incision superiorly. In addition, a scleral tunnel incision is naturally more rectangular, giving an extra margin of safety in closure and making suture closure, if necessary, more convenient in the scleral tissue rather than the more friable and difficult corneal location. Even if the corneal incision closes, it may well induce significant regular and irregular astigmatism.

Another convenient aspect of the blue line incision is the ability to enlarge the incision should the need arise for removing the lens or inserting a larger IOL (Figure 5-24). With a clear corneal incision, a separate scleral tunnel incision must be created to allow access with a larger incision. While this aspect of the blue line incision may be used infrequently, it is welcome when needed. We also believe that the scleral tissue absorbs phaco power, reducing wound healing and induced astigmatism from the phacoemulsification itself. A possible negative aspect of the incision is the possibility of developing chemosis during the surgery. If the surgery is efficient, this is rarely a problem and attention to the two points below can avoid it entirely. First, making a larger conjunctival opening than the proposed incision will usually prevent chemosis. We usually make a 4-mm opening for our 3-mm outer opening. Second, if chemosis begins to develop, simply opening the conjunctiva an additional amount will not only prevent further chemosis but will also make the chemosis that is present slowly resolve (Figures 5-25 and 5-26). A second cosmetic issue can be subconjunctival hemorrhage, which is unsightly and can usually be prevented with light cautery at the beginning and end of the case. We find that particular attention to the beginning and end of the conjunctival incision will control bleeding most effectively and additionally aid in wound closure at the end of the case. In cases with wound leakage at the end of the case, both hydration of the cornea and cautery at the ends of the incision will aid closure—an extra benefit of the blue line incision.

Figure 5-25. Photograph of the beginning of chemosis to the right of the phacoemulsification tip.

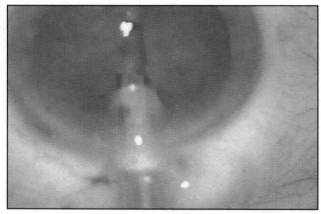

Figure 5-26. Photograph of the extension of the conjunctival opening to prevent further chemosis.

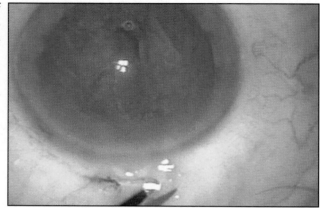

The final advantage of the blue line incision is seen in Figures 5-27 and 5-28. Here we see the appearance of the incision 1 week after surgery with excellent closure and virtually no possibility of leakage, even with an active lifestyle. Rapid recovery is dependent not only on vision but also on the ability to return to normal activities, both of which are facilitated by the blue line incision.

Results

In a prospective study, we examined the blue line incision by evaluating the postoperative astigmatic changes and the uncorrected visual acuity. A cohort of 364 cases was followed for at least 6 months. Postoperative data included uncorrected visual acuity, keratometric astigmatism, spherical equivalent, and corneal topography at each interval. Astigmatism analysis was based upon objective measurement according to keratometric readings. Changes in keratometric cylinder were evaluated by the simple subtraction method and the vector analysis described by Holladay, Koch, and Cravy.[10] Difference plots were performed on corneal topography between preoperative topography and postoperative measurements to assess induction of irregular astigmatism.

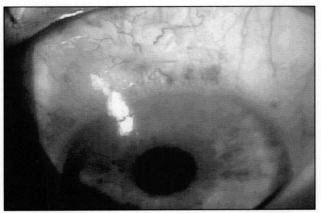

Figure 5-27. Slit lamp photograph of a blue line incision 1 week after surgery showing good wound healing and excellent closure.

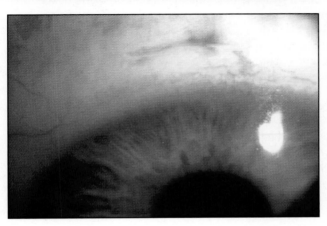

Figure 5-28. Slit lamp photograph of a blue line incision 1 week after surgery showing good wound healing and excellent closure.

Uncorrected Visual Acuity and Refractive Stability

Uncorrected visual acuity, especially at day 1, is a major parameter for assessing the efficacy and astigmatic neutrality of a self-sealing incision. This parameter is becoming one of the major postoperative criteria since cataract surgery is routinely performed ambulatory, through a small sutureless incision; thus, patients expect a fast visual recovery. In our study, 47% of the patients had uncorrected visual acuity of 20/40 or better at 1 day (Figure 5-29). At 3 and 6 months, 81% and 83% of the patients achieved an uncorrected visual acuity of 20/40 or better, respectively. The 1-day results of the blue line series appeared to be superior to the superior clear corneal ones. In fact, Grabow, et al found that at 1 day and 3 months postoperatively, only 35% and 60% of the patients were seeing 20/40 or better, respectively, with the superior clear corneal incision. This difference can be explained by the fact that superior clear corneal incisions are closer to the visual axis and therefore induce more astigmatism and are more likely a source of transient postoperative corneal edema. In fact, corneal edema at 1 day is seen more often and in more significant degrees with clear corneal incisions due to absorption of phaco power in the cornea and relative fluid incompetence of the wound as compared to the blue line incision. In these terms, the blue line incision enables a fast visual recovery with less corneal edema and quieter eyes. Higher percentages,

50%

Figure 5-29. Uncorrected vision at 1 day after blue line incision.

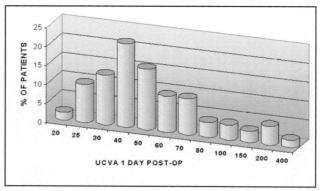

more comparable to the ones obtained with the blue line incision, were found by the same authors when the clear corneal incision was performed temporally. These results suggest that the clear corneal incision needs to be performed temporally to maximize the immediate postoperative visual recovery. This restriction can be considered a limit for surgeons who do not feel comfortable with the temporal approach of cataract incision. In addition, the temporal location (which will be discussed in the comparative section) is less appropriate than the superior location in terms of induced astigmatism.

Refractive stability was evaluated as a significant determinant of wound stability. In fact, changes in the astigmatic portion of the refraction can affect the spherical portion of the refraction and decrease the accuracy of the final refractive outcome. Mean spherical equivalent remained almost stable throughout the follow-up period with no significant differences at each interval—mean spherical equivalent –0.56 + 0.78 D at 1 month, -0.61 + 0.72 D at 3 months, and –0.57 + 0.78 D at 6 months (Figure 5-30).

Astigmatism

In cataract surgery, the incision must not be considered a simple entry port into the eye. In fact, the postoperative visual rehabilitation is primarily linked to the incision location, its architecture, and its construction; one of the most important factors that will influence the visual outcome is the postoperative astigmatism. The surgically induced astigmatism can be evaluated with two methods. First, the subtraction method, which calculates the absolute change between preoperative and postoperative keratometric astigmatism disregarding the axis component. Second, a vector analysis that evaluates not only the cylinder power but also the axis shift of the induced astigmatism. The final cylinder is the result of two obliquely crossed cylinders (preoperative and postoperative cylinders' powers with their axes). The surgically induced astigmatism with its axis is analyzed with a trigonometric solution. Vector methods are more appropriate to quantify the amount and the direction of cylinder induced by the surgery.

In our study, we evaluated the postoperative astigmatism with the two methods mentioned above. The vector analysis was performed according to the Koch, Holladay, and Cravy method. Figure 5-31 represents the mean preoperative and postoperative astigmatism evaluated with the simple subtraction method. Mean preoperative astigmatism was 0.96 + 0.68 D and postoperatively 0.99 + 0.76 D at 1 month, 0.89 + 0.64 D at 3 months, and 1 + 0.84 D at 6 months. The difference between preoperative and postoperative mean astigma-

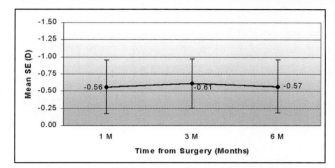

Figure 5-30. Average spherical equivalent shown over time showing stability of correction.

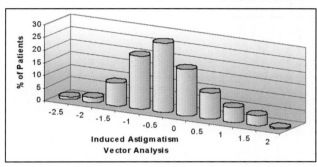

Figure 5-31. Induced vector astigmatic analysis comparing pre- and postoperative astigmatism.

tism at each interval is not statistically significant according to ANOVA analysis (P = 0.06). These results show that the blue line incision is astigmatically neutral, as we would expect from a scleral tunnel incision.

The astigmatic neutrality of the blue line incision is also proven by the results of the vector analysis, as shown in Figure 5-32. At each interval, mean surgically induced astigmatism was against the wound (negative values) and ranged from –0.47 + 0.50 D at 1 month to –0.57 + 0.40 D at 3 months and –0.52 + 0.43 D at 6 months. Mean surgically induced astigmatism was not statistically significant over the postoperative period (P = 0.47). The distribution of the surgically induced astigmatism is shown in Figure 5-33. Induced astigmatism was found to be neutral in 18% of the cases, against the wound in 60% of the cases including 27% within -0.50 D and 48% within -1 D. Figure 5-33 shows that 56% of the patients had a surgically induced astigmatism within +0.50 D, 84% within +1 D, and 99% within +2 D.

On review of preoperative and postoperative corneal topography plots, no evidence of induced irregular astigmatism was observed.

This study has demonstrated that the blue line incision, as we would expect from a scleral tunnel incision, is almost astigmatic neutral. In fact, the amount of postoperative astigmatism can be considered almost nonsignificant in light of the fact that the measurement of astigmatism can vary more than 0.5 D from day to day.

Safety

Clinical issues of safety include incidence of wound leakage and hyphema occurring in the immediate postoperative period. We noted no postoperative leaks from the main incision. The architecture of the blue line incision and especially its squared dimensions guar-

Figure 5-32. Astigmatic stability over time showing no statistical astigmatic drift.

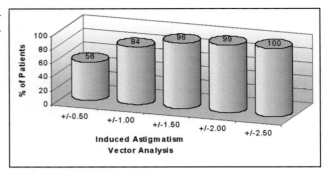

Figure 5-33. Induced vector astigmatic analysis comparing pre- and postoperative astigmatism.

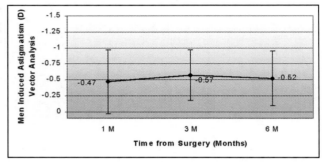

antees an excellent wound self-sealing. In our experience, wound hydration is rarely necessary to guarantee wound watertightness at the end of the procedure, whereas it occurs 25% more frequently with clear corneal incisions.

Loss of endothelial cells may also be included in the safety parameters. Grabow found a 13% cell loss in the superior corneal incision group compared to a 9% cell loss in the temporal corneal incision one.[11] This higher rate is linked to the fact that these incisions are closer to the central endothelium. In addition, the same author found in a comparative study between scleral pocket incisions and temporal clear corneal incisions, a linear relationship between ultrasound time and endothelial loss. When the ultrasound time varied from 0.5 to 1.5 minutes, the cell loss was comparable in both incision groups. However, beyond 1.5 minutes, the clear corneal incision cell loss rate appeared to be significantly higher than the scleral pocket one. In fact, beyond 3.5 and 4 minutes of ultrasound (U/S), the endothelial cell loss reached 14% and 28% in the corneal group, whereas the scleral pocket one only reached 6%. This information has clinical implications and may lead the surgeon to perform scleral incisions, especially in patients with advanced cataract or low preoperative endothelial cell counts.

Comparison of the Blue Line Incision With the Clear Corneal and Scleral Tunnel Incisions

The goal of the blue line incision is to combine the advantages of the clear corneal and the scleral tunnel incision (Tables 5-1 to 5-3). Scleral tunnel incisions have proven to be safe and stable, whereas clear corneal incisions were adopted for their efficiency. These past

Table 5-1

Clear Corneal Incision

+ Efficient
+ No bleeding
+ No cautery
- Not flexible
- Poor healing
- Higher astigmatism

Table 5-2

Scleral Tunnel Incision

+ Less induced astigmatism
+ Flexible
+ Wound healing
- Time consuming
- Bleeding
- Cautery

years, emphasis on reducing procedural time has become the dominant trend in cataract surgery. As such, clear corneal incisions have grown in popularity mainly because of their efficiency. In fact, clear corneal incisions do not require peritomy and cautery and thus can be quickly performed. In addition, clear corneal incisions enable the surgeon to perform cataract surgery under topical anesthesia. This concept of topical anesthesia and clear corneal incision is particularly seductive. It not only allows for an immediate visual rehabilitation but is more cost effective.[12] However, the emphasis should be primarily on quality and safety, not merely on efficiency. It is by no means certain that the shift of the external opening of the incision toward the cornea is beneficial. In fact, it is our contention that it is a negative development whose disadvantages are hidden by the smaller incision size routinely employed for clear corneal incisions. The blue line incision can be performed as fast as a clear corneal incision, as it does not require a peritomy. Moreover, the limited size of the incision does not induce significant bleeding and so requires only mild and superficial cautery, which has a limited impact in terms of astigmatism. Finally, topical anesthesia is not incompatible with the blue line incision or any other limbal or scleral sutureless incision as long as patient selection, wound construction, and phacoemulsification are properly performed.

In terms of safety, the blue line incision, as a square scleral tunnel incision, provides an excellent watertightness and wound healing. This statement has already been demonstrated in previous studies. In fact, Ernest has shown in his experimental studies that leakage occurred more frequently in rectangular shaped clear corneal incisions than in square scleral tunnel incisions.[13] Moreover, scleral tunnel incisions were more stable and more resistant to external pressure than clear corneal incisions. Finally, Ernest and Neuhann have shown

Table 5-3

Blue Line Incision

+ Less induced astigmatism
+ Flexible
+ Wound healing
+ Efficient
- Potential for bleeding
- Potential for chemosis

that incisions located in a vascular area healed in only 6 days, whereas clear corneal incisions needed up to 60 days.[9]

In terms of surgically induced astigmatism, several authors have shown that corneal incisions allow for limited induced astigmatism, fast visual recovery, and satisfactory refractive stability.[14,15,16] However, clear corneal incisions become less forgiving and may induce significantly more regular or irregular astigmatism and leakage in cases of construction imperfections. Gills and Sanders, based on Samuelson's cadaver study, described the relationship between the location of the external incision and the induced astigmatism.[17,18] The farther the incision is from the visual axis, the less induced astigmatism is promoted. Moreover, Koch studied the relationship between the induced astigmatism and the incision location and width.[19] If we consider the incisional funnel as defined by Koch, the 3.0 mm blue line incision by its location and width fits perfectly in the funnel and thus induces limited surgically induced astigmatism.

Olsen, et al[20] compared the induced regular and irregular astigmatism after sutureless scleral and corneal tunnel incision. In their study, 100 eyes underwent a 3.5 to 4.0 mm wide clear corneal or scleral tunnel incision performed in the steepest axis of the corneal astigmatism. The mean surgically induced astigmatism was computed by vector analysis for the two groups with a 6-month follow-up. One day after surgery, the surgically induced astigmatism was 1.41 D ± 0.66 (SD [standard deviation]) in the corneal incision group and 0.55 ± 0.31 (SD) in the scleral incision group. Six months after the surgery, the induced astigmatism was 0.72 ± 0.35 D and 0.36 ± 0.21 D, respectively. The differences in induced astigmatism were statistically significant and persisted over time. The astigmatism changes were confirmed by the corneal topography data. Moreover, Fourier harmonic series analysis of the topographic data showed significantly more irregular induced astigmatism in the clear corneal group. This study demonstrated that the clear corneal incision induces more regular and irregular astigmatism than does the scleral tunnel incision.

Joo, et al[21] also noted that the clear corneal incision induced significantly more flattening along the incisional meridian than the scleral tunnel incision. Their study retrospectively compared 6.0 mm scleral tunnel incisions to 3.1 mm clear corneal incisions. The changes in surgically induced astigmatism were evaluated with a computer-assisted videokeratography (CVK) at 1 day, and 2 and 6 months postoperatively. The CVK measurements showed more flattening at radial distances of 0.75, 1.50, and 2.50 mm along the 90-degree semimeridian in the clear corneal group, with narrower and longer flattening in the CVK pattern. The amount of flattening decreased at 8 weeks in all groups, and the differences between the groups became not statistically significant.

Special Techniques

Kurt A. Buzard, MD, FACS

Introduction

This chapter will present topics that do not neatly fit under other categories discussed in this book, or while of importance, do not merit a chapter of their own. Despite the frequent change of focus, the goal of this book is to assemble in one place a variety of techniques and instruments that might facilitate refractive phacoemulsification. Aside from the exact issues discussed here, we hope to show by specific examples in our practice, the attention to detail that can enhance 1-day uncorrected vision and the entire refractive experience for the patient. Refractive surgical patients represent a new challenge in ophthalmology, requiring not only a "good result," but the achievement of that result with comfort and speed. Issues that might have been considered superfluous only a few years ago are now seen as essential to the maintenance and growth of a refractive surgical practice. With this mindset, we would like to present the topics contained in this chapter.

Techniques for efficient removal of the lens have a great impact on the safety and short-term visual rehabilitation of the patient. It is, of course, always important to extract the lens without breaking the capsule, using excessive ultrasonic power, damaging endothelium, or, in general, being too rough to the eye while at the same time efficiently removing the lens. These matters assume even greater importance when clear lens exchange is performed. Breaking the capsule should be the rarest of events in this circumstance and the surgeon should be both experienced and sure of technique prior to moving to this refractive modality. In addition, the patient expectations are heightened with regard to rapid visual rehabilitation. Several issues are of interest and should be discussed. First, several techniques have been described to remove the lens, and although many share the same benefits and overall surgery time, they may not be equal in terms of safety, roughness of removal, or endothelial damage. Second, removal of a soft lens can be quite different than a firmer cataract; and even different densities of cataract can dictate technique. Techniques such as cracking and chopping[1–5] depend on splitting the nucleus and do not work at all in a soft lens. Even divide and conquer[2] needs to be modified since a soft human lens does not break but instead bends. In fact, the best methods for clear lens surgery rely on techniques that are applicable to cataract surgery only in a general sense. Chip and flip[3] is a technique that we have found particularly useful, especially if hydrodelineation is performed with a relatively small nuclear fragment. Its advantage is the ease with which the central portion of the lens can be lifted through a capsulorrhexis of approximately the same size while protecting the capsular bag with a thick layer of epinuclear material. Conversely, the technique for removing this thick epinuclear and cortex must be sure and without complication, as we will describe. Additionally, we find that a one-handed technique is superior in our hands since the second instrument is not used for chopping or cracking[1,5] and, in fact, can get in the way of surgery. We have also found a variant of divide and conquer that can provide an efficient and useful method of removal, which we will discuss later in the chapter.

Of utmost importance is the careful consideration of the time for visual rehabilitation. This is always an issue but assumes even more importance when treating the refractive patient. Thus, a timeframe for visual recovery that may be acceptable for a cataract patient may be completely unacceptable when dealing with a refractive patient. One day postoperative vision assumes importance as a pathway to rapid visual function in everyday activities. The choice of incision should result in a strong closure with minimal edema and little, if no, discomfort. Elsewhere in this book we discuss the suitability of the blue line incision in terms of each of these requirements. The cosmetic appearance of the eye is equally important and one should avoid hemorrhage from the incision and/or unnecessary roughness on the globe. When performing the phacoemulsification, it is preferable to primarily use suction, although excessive time in the eye may diminish 1-day postoperative vision, and light bursts of ultrasound may be appropriate. For both cataract surgery and lens exchange, fluid washing through the eye across unprotected endothelial cells will encourage corneal edema[6–8] that will in turn reduce early postoperative visual acuity. To help discourage this, liberal use of viscoelastic[9–13] will coat the endothelial cells and protect them from damage. This covering can be easily displaced by rough maneuvers within the eye or by excessive time in the eye, allowing the viscoelastic protection to be washed away. Therefore, while care to avoid complications is imperative, it is equally important to avoid excess time in the eye. Additionally, while viscoelastic protection is beneficial during the surgery, it is vital that it be removed at the conclusion of the case, since a pressure rise the night of the surgery will certainly compromise uncorrected visual acuity the next day, and even worse, cause the patient discomfort. All of these points are well known and yet need to be emphasized again. Later in this chapter we will discuss these points with small techniques that may assist the completeness or speed with which they are accomplished.

When performing surgery for refractive purposes, each detail needs to be reexamined, whether it be the comfort of the patient before and during surgery, surgical technique, or postoperative care. Perhaps one of the most important aspects of the development of a refractive lens-based practice is the care of the patient before and after surgery. Refractive patients demand a different level of care, and long-held practices might well need to be examined with respect to these needs. It is not always disagreeable to change, in fact many changes are long overdue and pertain to common sense practice. These procedures may already be in place but may need to be enhanced, particularly with respect to the mindset of the staff. In the past, specifics of medical care were often unknown to the patient, or at the least a subject that was discussed only face-to-face with the physician. Today, patients are well-educated and frequently have reasonable questions with respect to their problem and the cost of resolving it. While staff cannot replace a personal evaluation and discussion with the surgeon, they can set the tone for the coming visit; the more knowledgeable and courteous they are, the more comfortable the patient will be in the upcoming evaluation. It is amazing how a single untoward remark or unkind response can lead to a wary patient and an unsatisfactory consultation. Staff members, particularly those answering the phones, must be included in changes in refractive orientation and procedures and should be given scripts for common questions. Areas of specific concern, such as complications or unrealistic expectations, should not be avoided, but every attempt should be made to refer such calls to a counselor or coordinator within the practice who can deal with such issues in more detail. Above all, common sense questions should be known by all and if the discussion leads to an area in which the staff member is unsure, the response should be that the person does not know the answer but will quickly and courteously transfer the patient to someone who does. With the advent of the Internet and numerous self-help television and popular press articles, patients are often well-educated and articulate in their need for information and will not accept the answer that these questions will be addressed in the visit. For this reason, we now believe that the position of patient counselor or coordinator is necessary for all but the smallest practices. This "face" of the practice must be constantly refined and evaluated. It is not unwise to periodically call your own practice and put yourself in the place of the patient to decide for yourself if the presentation is what you desire.

Patient expectations represent the next important issue prior to proposed surgery, and if carefully addressed, can lead to uneventful and pleasant postoperative visits; but if poorly or inadequately presented, they can represent problems even in a "good" result. Issues revolving about the difference between reading and distance vision can be a potential source of trouble. Even a patient with 20/20 uncorrected distance correction may be dissatisfied if the problem of poor close vision is not discussed prior to the procedure. While such complaints may have been dismissed in the past, they must be addressed as an area of "new thinking." We utilize "monovision" as a primary modality to address reading issues and will try contact lenses whenever possible prior to surgery to allow a demonstration of the idea. For patients in their 40s, a monovision correction of -1.50 to -1.75 diopters (D) is acceptable, but patients in their 50s and older frequently ask for more correction, in the range of -2.00 to -2.25 D. Rather than testing eye dominance, we will ask the simple question, "Which eye would you sight a camera or telescope with?" We find this method much more successful than objective testing. If possible, we will attempt a contact lens trial for a few days to a week to ensure a positive response to the correction and find a high acceptance rate. We are careful to point out that monovision is not perfect and that for night driving and/or extended reading, additional correction may be required. We are also careful to have a consistent and careful discussion of the benefits and problems with monovision, including the pleasures of reading one's watch, working on a computer, and enhanced up and down vision. We find this encourages acceptance and places this technique in a realistic context. Surprisingly, we find that as the patients move out of the work force and enter their 60s and 70s, the trend is against monovision, and in fact when performed, the patients often refer to the near eye as their "bad" eye. For this reason we move toward bilateral distance vision as a rule in this age group. These patients do not mind simple reading glasses, and we are careful to recommend them on the first postoperative day, as many patients do not realize these will work for them after surgery. As an alternative, for those patients who find monovision unacceptable, we offer the Array (Allergan, Irvine, Calif) multifocal intraocular lens in selected cases. While the number of cases is small (about 5% in our practice), we find this to be a benefit in some patients; this alternative is discussed in more detail elsewhere in this book. Again, careful discussion of the benefits and problems are essential to proper patient acceptance of this lens. In all discussions, we point out the possibility of lens exchange should the patient be dissatisfied, and we are not slow to replace the lens when problems arise.

A general idea of the number and purpose of the postoperative visits is helpful. Many patients lead busy lives and do not wish to be burdened by unnecessary and/or lengthy visits, sometimes remembering past times in which parents underwent lengthy recuperation from cataract surgery. We routinely separate surgeries on the two eyes by a week or less and inform the patient that a return to normal activities is usually possible the next day and that it is not unusual to perform surgery on consecutive days. The purpose of the first postoperative visit is self evident but also provides an opportunity to evaluate astigmatic and spherical error and to correct these in selected instances. For pre-existing against-the-rule astigmatism, we will perform slit lamp astigmatic surgery on the first postoperative visit and will often see an improvement in uncorrected vision from 20/50 or worse to 20/25 or 20/30 with the application of artificial tears. If a spherical error is present in the operated eye or contralateral eye, disposable soft contact lenses will be placed to facilitate return to normal activities.

Most patients are independent, need to drive, are often working, and even a small delay in visual rehabilitation can be a significant downside to the surgery. This is in distinction to cataract surgery in the past, when the patient was ferried to and from appointments and visual recovery could be delayed as long as 2 to 3 months, often with almost as long a wait to do surgery on the other eye. Those days are long gone, and each day in which the patient cannot drive or function will be attributed to a poor result; while prompt recovery will be reported to friends and colleagues as proof that the surgery is a success.

We routinely see the patient at 1 day and 2 weeks, during which time the vision is adjusted if necessary with relaxing incisions and postoperative medications are given. We will then see the patient in 2 to 3 months if no further issues are present. If a spherical error is present, we will see the patient in 2 to 4 weeks and schedule a lens exchange (intraocular lens [IOL] exchanged to proper power based on refraction only). We find no benefit in waiting more than 6 weeks, since the refraction rarely changes significantly after that time. At the 2-week visit, we educate the patient concerning the need for follow-up if vision changes and there is a possibility of capsular opacification in the future, which can be treated on the same day with YAG laser capsulotomy. If the patient is a myope, we emphasize the need to recognize the importance of flashes and floaters. As much as possible, patient visits are kept to a minimum and things are done in a single visit (such as YAG capsulotomy) rather than waste the patient's time with multiple visits. All of this is in keeping with the need to treat the patient exactly as a refractive patient is treated and to make the number of surprises minimal and the postoperative course simple.

Preoperative Patient Care

For surgeons familiar with refractive surgical procedures such as laser-assisted in situ keratomileusis (LASIK), the preparation of the patient for surgery is well known. To review, the better educated the patient in regard to the procedure and its inherent risks, the better the experience will be for both surgeon and patient. Issues that may or may not be discussed with a cataract patient should be discussed in detail with the potential refractive exchange patient. Some of the issues we discuss are:

- Transportation to and from the facility
- The method of anesthesia
- What the patient can expect to feel during surgery and afterward
- The noises that he or she may hear during surgery

- Specific numbers concerning the outcome with respect to vision
- The percentages and types of potential complications

In addition, we discuss the percentage of chance for enhancement, and how and when that surgical procedure occurs (specifically with respect to relaxing incisions, lens exchange, and even LASIK). One subject that is frequently left undiscussed is the potential for YAG laser capsulotomy, why the clouding of the capsule occurs, and the simplicity of treatment. We perform both relaxing incisions and YAG laser on the date of the diagnostic visit so as to reduce the inconvenience of additional visits and anxiety concerning these procedures. The consent process is the same as for cataract surgery, but it is particularly important to point out that no guarantees are given with respect to uncorrected vision. Again with respect to cosmetic issues, we also have the patient sign a statement that ptosis may occur after surgery.

As with any surgical procedure, we ask the patient to present on the day of surgery in loose-fitting clothing without makeup and have the patient wash his or her face with Phisohex (Bayer, Myerstown, Pa) prior to surgery. Our use of an intravenous (IV) line has been limited. In our experience, patients complained of discomfort from the IV more than any other aspect of the operation. Therefore, we do not routinely employ an IV except in patients with cardiac or respiratory illness, and instead utilize Xanax (Pharmacia & Upjohn, Peapack, NJ) 0.5 mg orally to reduce anxiety and promote patient comfort. Materials to start an IV are kept in all patient areas, but since moving away from IV 2 years ago, we have rarely had a need to start an IV line. We observed one reaction in which the patient appeared to develop an allergic response to the medication with extrapyrimidal symptoms. The reaction resolved completely about 1 hour after transfer to the hospital. No technique is completely safe, but these steps have significantly contributed to the overall comfort of the patient.

Along the same lines, many patients object to oxygen given through the nasal cannula. Instead, we have found that a device that both lifts the drapes away from the patient's face and provides oxygen is more comfortable and results in fewer complaints (Figures 6-1a and b).

Surgical Techniques, Instruments, and Materials

The prevention of complications is a priority in any surgery and expectations are heightened when performing refractive surgery. One complication of particular importance is infection and/or endophthalmitis. The use of preoperative topical antibiotics has been described and varies in use from 3 or 4 days prior to surgery to just drops in the waiting room. To be effective, it is preferable to have aqueous levels of antibiotic prior to surgery.[14] The problem is that almost immediately the antibiotic concentration rapidly diminishes so that any direct ocular application of the antibiotic is probably lost. Use of antibiotics in the irrigation solution has also been described, particularly Vancomycin, although this too can pose a problem since the amount of medication may be too high during the case and may be overly diluted at the end when refilling the eye. Additionally, the use of Vancomycin poses a public health problem if endophthalmitis occurs, as it will be resistant to Vancomycin; and the widespread use of Vancomycin will encourage the emergence of these bacteria. Many hospitals have banned the routine use of Vancomycin for just this reason.

The choice of incision is also important, and endophthalmitis has been associated with poorly closed clear corneal incisions, as referenced by Maurice John, MD, in this book. It is

Figure 6-1a. Striker oxygen delivery tube showing position of patient head, providing oxygen and maintaining separation of the drape.

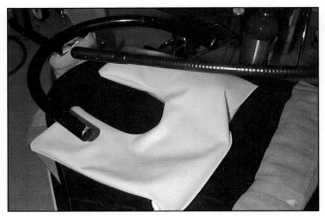

Figure 6-1b. Striker oxygen delivery tube showing position of patient head, providing oxygen and maintaining separation of the drape.

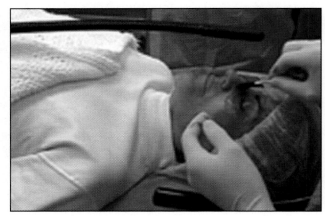

for this reason that we use the blue line incision since we have had no cases of endophthalmitis in several thousand cases with no wound leaks.

The most effective single treatment to prevent endophthalmitis is the use of diluted Betadine (Perdue Frederick, Norwalk, Conn) solution in the cul-de-sac prior to surgery.[14–17] We prepare the patient with Betadine solution on the skin and eyelids prior to surgery and do not scrub the lashes. We believe this presents more bacteria from secretions of the meibomian glands than are eradicated by the scrubbing. We dry the skin and utilize Steristrips (3M, St. Paul, Minn) to open the eye prior to the application of an adherent plastic barrier (Figure 6-2a). Failure to dry the skin will result in shifting drapes and a greater risk of contamination. We then create an incision in the drape that allows excess plastic material to "wrap" the lashes, removing them from the surgical field (Figures 6-2b and c). At the conclusion of surgery, we use what we believe to be the second most effective treatment against endophthalmitis: subconjunctival injections of antibiotic adjacent to the incision (Figure 6-3). We use cefazolian 50 mg/ml, gentimycin 40 mg/ml, and celestone all mixed in the same syringe and given in a quantity of approximately of 0.5 cc with the remainder washed over the surface of the eye. This deposit of antibiotics will gradually release over a 24-hour period and provide a powerful resistance to endophthalmitis. In the thousands of intraocular cases that I have performed in my career, I have never had an endophthalmitis associated

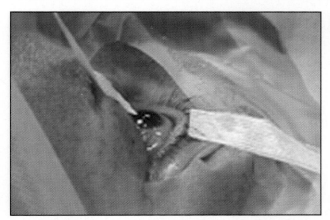

Figure 6-2a. Use of Steristrips to maintain lid opening prior to use of a plastic drape.

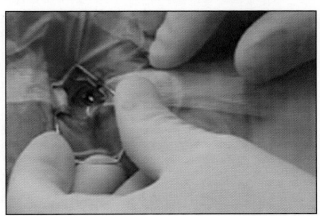

Figure 6-2b. Wrapping of drape material around the lids and lashes to isolate these areas from the surgical field.

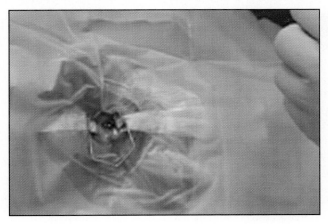

Figure 6-2c. Final appearance of draping with plastic material wrapped around the lids.

with a subconjunctival injection of antibiotics. Since the incidence of endophthalmitis is low,[19–22] this alone does not constitute proof, but I believe the rationale is appropriate, as I do not use antibiotics in my irrigating solution nor do I use antibiotic drops.

Once draped, we perform a blue line incision on the eye, approximately 2.5 mm wide on the inside of the tunnel, as described elsewhere in this book. We prefer a relatively small

Figure 6-3. Appearance of subconjunctival injection of antibiotics at the conclusion of a case.

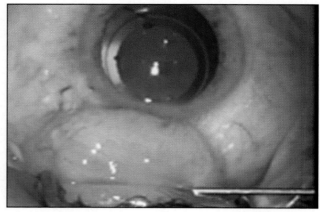

Figure 6-4. Chang cannula (No 15-20-CHG) (Mastel Precision).

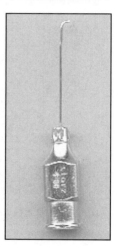

capsulorrhexis, approximately 5 mm in diameter, which we use with a STAAR (Monrovia, Calif) IOL that then overlaps the optic and maintains the lens iris diaphragm, holding the vitreous in place. As we have discussed elsewhere in this book, the use of a small capsulor-rhexis with a small YAG laser capsulotomy can be a deterrent to retinal detachment in the future. We use a Chang cannula (No 15-20-CHG) (Mastel Precision) that allows better control of hydrodissection (Figure 6-4). With the short right-angle tip, the surgeon is able to direct fluid orthogonally to the edge of the lens nearly 365 degrees, providing a more rapid and complete hydrodissection. This allows easier subsequent hydrodissection of the nucleus and better control in cleaving different planes in a soft lens, as we discussed above. We routinely cleave two plains for a soft lens, creating one plane with the epinucleus and a thick cortex to protect the capsule. We then hydrodissect more peripherally to facilitate later removal of the cortex (Figure 6-5). The use of vigorous hydrodissection coupled with the subsequent gentle downward central pressure with the cannula will both facilitate later surgery and create a good cleavage plane.

We utilize two basic techniques for removal of the nucleus, both one-handed and used together. The first is a variant of chip and flip, in which we carve (with minimal use of ultra-sound) a central grove extending through the outside edge of the nucleus. We then extend

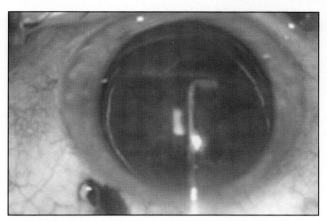

Figure 6-5. Creation of hydrodelineation with a small nuclear fragment and a larger hydrodissection showing a "golden ring."

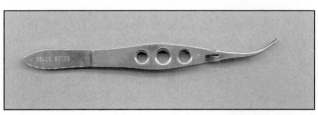

Figure 6-6. Salz cracking forceps (Solos S7729).

the central grove in a fan shape to the right and left, removing the majority of the soft nucleus. With a single 180-degree rotation, the remainder of the nucleus is engaged and will rotate upward out of the capsulorrhexis, allowing completion of the removal of the soft nucleus.

When removing an actual cataract or a lens that is slightly more firm, we have found that a one-handed technique utilizing the divide and conquer method with the Salz cracking forceps (Solos S7729, Norcross, Ga) can be more efficient and will require fewer rotations of the nucleus, resulting in less opportunity for complications (Figure 6-6). In this technique, a deep central grove is made within the confines of the capsulorrhexis and viscoelastic is introduced into the chamber. The cracking forceps are used to create the first cracking plane (Figures 6-7a and b) and the nucleus is then rotated 90 degrees. It is then possible to create another deep grove within the confines of the capsulorrhexis on both halves of the nucleus. Again, with the introduction of viscoelastic, the nucleus may be divided into four pieces. Each piece is then removed in the usual manner with the phacoemulsification probe.

The advantage of this technique over traditional two-handed cracking and/or chopping techniques is in the relative time irrigation is used in the eye and in the safety of the procedure. The endothelium is recoated twice during the procedure and is thus protected while the cracking with the forceps is performed—unlike two-handed techniques in which the cracking and subsequent removal are part of one continuous process. Additionally, very complete cleavage is obtained with minimal downward pressure and only one 90-degree rotation of the nucleus, resulting in greater capsular safety. Because the forces of the cross-action Salz forceps are directed perfectly against the sides of the grove, a complete opening is made with minimal trauma, which is difficult to do with a two-handed technique. This again facilitates and shortens the time required to remove the remaining nuclear material. While many other efficient and safe methods exist to remove the nucleus, we find that this

Figure 6-7a. Insertion of Salz cracking forceps with viscoelastic in place.

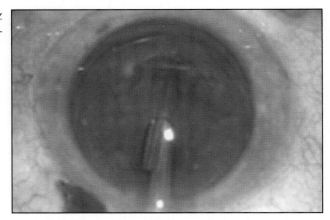

Figure 6-7b. Opening of forceps showing a crack developing centrally.

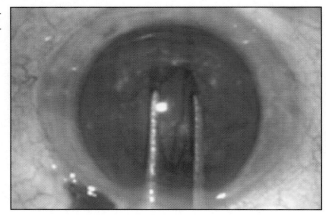

technique minimizes phaco time, irrigation time, and total surgical time. One technique that we have found particularly useful in terms of phacoemulsification is to centrally swirl the tip of the phacoemulsifier to encourage aspiration of the nuclear material. In addition, we attempt to engage in aspirating the nucleus at or below the plane of the anterior capsule to minimize endothelial trauma. To this end, we will often remove additional nuclear material after cracking before removing the nuclear fragments to minimize phaco trauma in a very hard nucleus.

The second technique for a soft lens in clear lens surgery involves a variant of divide and conquer, in which a deep grove is created extending through the edge of the nucleus (Figure 6-8a). The lens is then rotated 90 degrees (Figure 6-8b), and a second deep grove is made through the edge of the nucleus, creating one-quarter of the nucleus with only a thin adherence to the remainder by the thinned bottom of the groves (Figure 6-8c). This fragment is then engaged and removed from the nucleus by tearing along the previous groves (Figure 6-8d). With this section gone, the soft nucleus is compressible, and if one end is engaged (Figure 6-8e), it can be delivered through the capsulorrhexis in one piece and removed with the phaco tip as it is being delivered (Figure 6-8f).

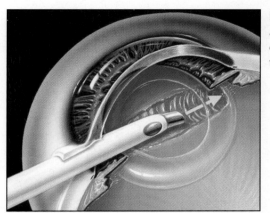

Figure 6-8a. Illustration of the divide and conquer variant for a soft nucleus. A deep grove is created extending through the edge of the nucleus.

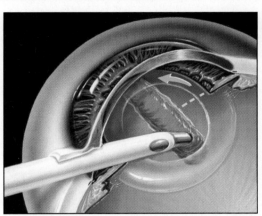

Figure 6-8b. The lens is then rotated 90 degrees.

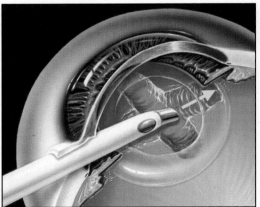

Figure 6-8c. A second deep grove is made through the edge of the nucleus, creating one-quarter of the nucleus with only a thin adherence to the remainder by the thinned bottom of the groves.

Figure 6-8d. The fragment is then engaged and removed from the nucleus by tearing along the previous groves.

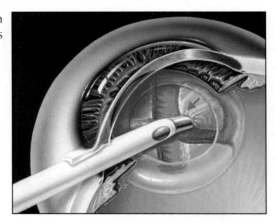

Figure 6-8e. The nucleus is rotated and engaged.

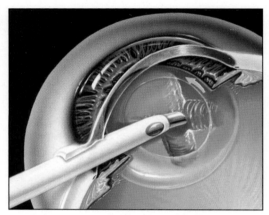

Figure 6-8f. The nucleus can then be delivered through the capsulorrhexis in one piece and removed with the phaco tip as it is being delivered.

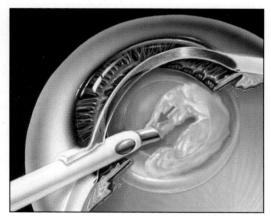

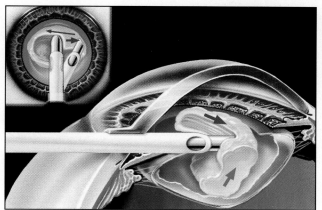

Figure 6-9a. Illustration of the first step of thick epinuclear and cortex removal in which the bevel is turned downward and the cortex is engaged at 6 o'clock. The tip is withdrawn slightly and, by moving side to side, the material is aspirated.

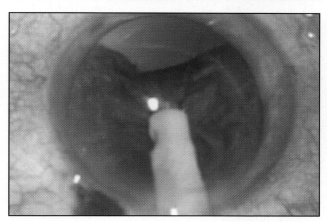

Figure 6-9b. Photograph of the first step of thick epinuclear and cortex removal in which the bevel is turned downward and the cortex is engaged at 6 o'clock. The tip is withdrawn slightly and, by moving side to side, the material is aspirated.

Swipe and Swallow

Once the nuclear material is removed, we immediately begin removal of cortex with the phaco tip. With the large phaco tip opening, it is much easier to remove a thick cortical coating that otherwise might break off in pieces, making aspiration with the irrigation/aspiration (I/A) tip difficult or impossible. We have named this technique "swipe and swallow" to illustrate the dynamic nature of the procedure and to illustrate the efficiency of the procedure with the name. Again, application of the phaco tip for aspiration is much quicker and reduces total irrigation time within the eye, enhancing postoperative visual recovery. The technique involves engaging the cortex at 6 o'clock and maintaining a back and forth motion. It is important to maintain movement of the phaco tip at all times since if the tip remains stationary, the capsule will be naturally drawn to it and may be ruptured. We face the bevel downward and engage the cortex at 6 o'clock (Figures 6-9a and b). The tip is moved back and forth and as this motion occurs, cortex enters the tip and is sheared by the sides of the tip, gradually removing the cortex material. The tip should be maintained in the plane of the anterior capsule, making the cortex peel upward away from the capsule and gradually removing the cortical "shield" (Figures 6-10a and b). As long as the phaco tip is full of cortical material, the capsule is safe, but if the surgeon allows the tip to clear, the cap-

Figure 6-10a. Illustration of the second portion of thick cortex removal in which the tip is moved from side to side in the plane of the anterior capsule, drawing the material upward and shearing it off in thin ribbons that are then aspirated.

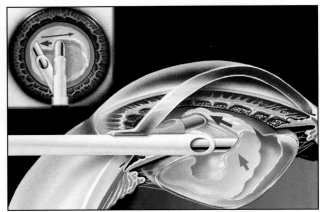

Figure 6-10b. Photo of the second portion of thick cortex removal in which the tip is moved from side to side in the plane of the anterior capsule, drawing the material upward and shearing it off in thin ribbons that are then aspirated.

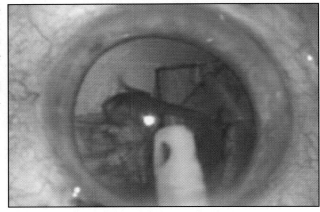

sule may be drawn upward. For this reason, the technique is best performed with a thick epinucleus. If a thin layer of cortex is remaining, it may be best to simply use the I/A tip. As the phaco tip goes to each side, it is rotated slightly and the material under the capsulorrhexis is engaged for another pass through the center. In relatively quick fashion, almost the entire cortex can be removed with the exception of the portion directly beneath the wound. Sometimes even the portion of cortex beneath the wound may be removed by engaging the remaining cortex and moving the tip away from the wound (Figures 6-11a and b). In many cases, this final maneuver is not possible and should not be attempted due to danger of capsular rupture. No more than 10 to 15 seconds are required for cortical removal with this method. The superior cortex can then be removed with the I/A tip, beginning on one side and with a sideways motion moving to the opposite side of the remaining cortex, which in many cases will be peeled from the capsule in one piece (Figure 6-12). The cortex is then aspirated in the iris plane with the opening pointed upward, without the need for a second instrument. As with the phaco tip, one good strategy to avoid capsular rupture is to constantly keep the tip of the I/A handpiece in motion, preferably along the edge of the anterior capsulorrhexis, thus removing cortex in larger pieces. In addition, peeling the cortex from the top down leaves fewer remnant fibers than peeling from the bottom up and requires less polishing of the capsule in the subsequent phase of the operation.

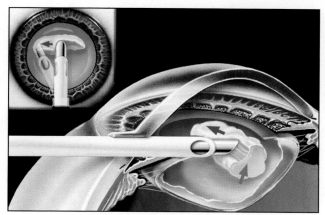

Figure 6-11a. Illustration of removal of the final portion of thick cortex with the phaco tip when possible. The material is engaged and the tip is extended away from the incision, allowing the remainder of cortex to break free and roll into the phaco tip.

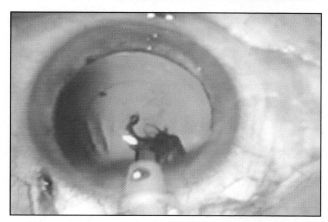

Figure 6-11b. Photo of removal of the final portion of thick cortex with the phaco tip when possible. The material is engaged and the tip is extended away from the incision, allowing the remainder of cortex to break free and roll into the phaco tip.

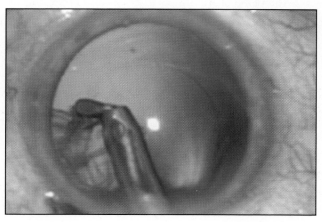

Figure 6-12. Photo of the small amount of residual cortex left for aspiration with the I/A tip.

One final useful technique is polishing of the anterior capsule. After insertion of the intraocular lens and before removal of the viscoelastic is an opportune moment to polish the debris located on the anterior capsule. We have found the polishing rings designed by Shepherd (Morning/STAAR MH-1433) to be helpful in removing the haze on the anterior capsule, which commonly occurs at the end of the case (Figure 6-13). With the viscoelastic

Figure 6-13. Shepherd polishing rings (Morning/ STAAR MH-1433).

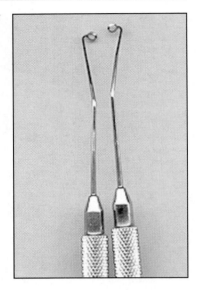

in place, the anterior chamber is kept well formed; and with both right and left polishers, it is possible to polish virtually the entire capsule in a short period of time, again with little or no endothelial trauma (Figure 6-14). Additionally, the posterior capsule is protected by the intraocular lens. Posterior capsular opacification is a matter of significant importance, and by polishing the capsule, we can decrease its incidence. In addition to the anterior capsule, posterior capsule polishing is important and we perform this maneuver prior to inserting the lens, as do most surgeons. Removal of the viscoelastic is extremely important in preventing postoperative intraocular pressure rise. It is also important to remove the viscoelastic beneath the lens. We use a technique in which the 45-degree tip of the I/A unit is directed downward with the irrigation ports in the plane of the intraocular lens and rotate the tip back and forth, which directs fluid beneath the iris and into the capsule, encouraging out-flow of viscoelastic. In addition, the lens can be moved back and forth with the I/A tip to further encourage egress of the viscoelastic material. If all of the material is removed, fine folds in the posterior capsule will be observed (Figure 6-15). If these folds are not observed, further irrigation/aspiration should be performed. On occasion, we will introduce the irriga-tion cannula beneath the lens to further irrigate and remove viscoelastic material. Careful attention to detail at this stage of the operation can virtually eliminate postoperative intraocular rise.

Conclusion

This chapter has covered a disparate number of topics, all focused on the small issues that contribute to decreased ultrasonic time, irrigation time, total operative time, and decreased trauma to the eye and endothelium. To achieve a high percentage of 1-day uncorrected 20/40 or better results, it is essential to concentrate on each aspect of the surgery. While many of the techniques and concepts presented here are common sense and are performed by other surgeons, the cumulative total of these techniques is to present a new focus for cataract and lens exchange surgery. Just as obtaining good uncorrected vision is a focus of

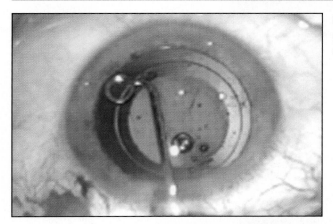

Figure 6-14. Use of Shepherd polishing forceps to clean anterior capsule debris.

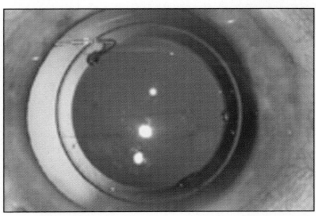

Figure 6-15. Posterior capsular fold seen when all viscoelastic has been removed.

refractive surgery, so too should be attention to patient comfort, safety, and the speed of visual recovery. Refractive phacoemulsification is not a new technique, rather it requires a state of mind willing to make changes to achieve better uncorrected vision in less time and with greater patient comfort and safety.

References

1. Ram J, Wesendahl TA, Auffarth GU, Apple DJ. Evaluation of in situ fracture versus phaco chop technique. *J Cataract Refract Surg.* 1998;24(11):1464-8.
2. Gimbel HV. Divide and conquer nucleofractis phacoemulsification: development and variations. *J Cataract Refract Surg.* 1991;17(3):281-91.
3. Kosrirukvongs P, Slade SG, Berkeley RG. Corneal endothelial changes after divide and conquer versus chip and flip phacoemulsification. *J Cataract Refract Surg.* 1997;23(7):1006-12.
4. Fine IH. The chip and flip phacoemulsification technique. *J Cataract Refract Surg.* 1991;17(3):366-71.
5. Koch PS, Katzen LE. Stop and chop phacoemulsification. *J Cataract Refract Surg.* 1994;20(5):566-70.

6. Bourne WM, Waller RR, Liesegang TJ, Brubaker RF. Corneal trauma in intracapsular and extracapsular cataract extraction with lens implantation. *Arch Ophthalmol.* 1981;99:1375-76.

7. Rao GN, Stevens RE, Harris JK, Aquavella JV. Long-term changes in corneal endothelium following intraocular lens implantation. *Ophthalmology.* 1981;88(5):386-97.

8. Oxford Cataract Treatment and Evaluation Team. Long-term corneal endothelial cell loss after cataract surgery. *Arch Ophthalmol.* 1986;104:1170-1175.

9. Pape LG, Balazs EA. The use of sodium hyaluronate (Healon) in human anterior segment surgery. *Ophthalmology.* 1980;87(7):699-705.

10. Miller D, Stegmann R. Use of Na-hyaluronate in anterior segment eye surgery (editorial). *Am Intra Ocular Implant Soc J.* 1980;6:13-15.

11. Miller D, Stegmann R. Use of sodium hyaluronate in human IOL implantation. *Ann Ophthalmol.* 1981;13:811-815.

12. Philipsson B, Holmberg A. Extracapsular cataract extraction by phacoemulsification using Healon. In: Miller D, Stegmann R, eds. *Healon (Sodium Hyaluronate): A Guide to its Uses in Ophthalmic Surgery.* New York, NY: John Wiley & Sons; 1983; 59-68.

13. Alpar JJ. Viscosurgery: a review of materials, indications, techniques, and precautions: In: Eisner G, ed. *Ophthalmic Viscosurgery.* Montreal, Quebec: Medicopea International Inc; 1986: 39-53.

14. Adenis JP, Robert PY, Mounier M, Denis F. Anterior chamber concentrations of Vancomycin in the irrigating solution at the end of cataract surgery. *J Cataract Refract Surg.* 1997;23(1):111-4.

15. Gills JP. Effective concentration of Betadine. *J Cataract Refract Surg.* 1999;25(5):604.

16. Isenberg DJ, Yoshimori R, Chang A, Lam GC, Wachler B, Neumann D. The effect of povidine-iodine solution applied at the conclusion of ophthalmic surgery. *Am J Ophthalmol.* 1996;119(6):701-5.

17. Caldwell DR, Kastl PR, Cook J, Simon J. Povidine-iodine: its efficacy as a preoperative conjunctival and periocular preparation.

18. Speaker MG, Menikoff JA. Prophylaxis of endophthalmitis with topical povidine-iodine. *Ophthalmology.* 1991;98(12):1796-75.

19. Morlet N, Gatus B, Coroneo M. Patterns of perioperative prophylaxis for cataract surgery: a survey of Australian ophthalmologists. *Aust N Z J Ophthalmol.* 1998;26(1):5-12.

20. Schmitz S, Dick HB, Krummenauer F, Pfeiffer N. Endophthalmitis in cataract surgery: results of a German survey. *Ophthalmology.* 1999;106(10):1869-77.

21. Liesegang TJ. Prophylactic antibiotics in cataract operations. *Mayo Clinic Proc.* 1997;72(2):149-59.

22. Adenis JP, Robert PY, Mounier M, Denis F. Anterior chamber concentrations of Vancomycin in the irrigating solution at the end of cataract surgery. *J Refract Surg.* 1997;23(1):111-4.

Astigmatism and Lens Extraction

Miles H. Friedlander, MD, FACS
Nicole S. Granet, BA
Luis E. Remus, PhD, MD
Lee H. Novick, MD

Either deliberately or unintentionally, ophthalmic surgeons who perform refractive cataract surgery, clear lens exchange, and multifocal intraocular lens implantation convey the promise of emmetropia to their patients. Patients who undergo conventional cataract extraction or corneal transplantation generally assume that they will be wearing glasses postoperatively, whereas refractive surgery patients are encouraged to believe that their reliance on optical correction will be greatly reduced or totally eliminated. The surgeon is thus committing him or herself to a procedure for which the end point is the elimination of refractive error. Critical to this assumption is the precise determination of the power of the intraocular lens. Accurate calculation requires precise A-scan readings to produce the desired spherical correction (see Chapter 11).

If one of the objectives of clear lens exchange is to permanently change the refractive error, we must have some idea of the refraction stability after several years. We reviewed the records of 43 patients who underwent cataract extraction by the same surgeon (Delmar Caldwell, MD) during 1992 to 1993. The operative technique was identical in all surgical candidates. Incision length was 6 mm and the pseudophakic lenses were all of the same model from the same manufacturer. One or two nylon sutures were used to close the surgical wound. We evaluated the refraction at 1 month, 1 year, and 5 years postoperatively. While the technique used was not small-incision sutureless surgery, if these wounds were stable over a 5-year period then it is safe to infer that wounds half the size (should) will also be stable. We examined sphere, cylinder power, and spherical equivalent for the postoperative periods of 1 month, 1 year, and 5 years. As refractive stability was the point of interest, this study does not address the question of accuracy of refraction—desired or final.

Table 7-1 summarizes the findings for postoperative sphere, cylinder, and spherical equivalent for the indicated periods.

Linear regression studies of these data comparing these measures shows the greatest correlation with the spherical equivalent. When comparing the entire data set for the postoperative period of 1 month and 1 year, the spherical equivalent had a correlation of 0.584. When comparing the 1-year and 5-year postoperative periods, the correlation had a modest improvement to 0.63. Comparison of the 1-month and 5-year postoperative periods demonstrated a correlation of 0.71. A careful review of the data revealed several outlying points. When these outlying data points were removed from the data set, the correlation for each of these time periods of comparison improved to approximately 0.8 for each comparison.

Table 7-1

Average Sphere, Cylinder, and Spherical Equivalent for 1 Month, 1 Year, and 5 Years

Refraction	1 Month (mean ± SEM)	1 Year (mean ± SEM)	5 Years (mean ± SEM)
Sphere	-1.13 ± 0.14 D	-1.15 ± 0.15 D	-1.33 ± 0.15 D
Cylinder	0.83 ± 0.09 D	0.97 ± 0.121 D	1.06 ± 0.12 D
Spherical equivalent	-0.71 ± 0.13 D	-0.67 ± 0.14 D	-0.82 ± 0.14 D

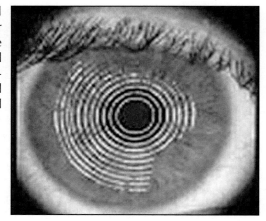

Figure 7-1. Left side of photo: normal photokeratoscope (PKS). The circular white lines are clear and sharp. The spaces between the lines are smooth and even. Right side of photo: irregular astigmatism. The white lines are irregular and uneven. Spaces between are angulated and vary in width.

Equally critical is the manipulation of the wound to eliminate or reduce preexisting astigmatism. Certainly, the wound must not induce undesirable astigmatism. The recent use of small-incision cataract surgery with or without sutures influences astigmatism very little. However, before the advent of small-incision cataract surgery with foldable intraocular lenses, wound size was an important factor in final astigmatic correction.[1] Incisions greater than 5.5 mm tended to decay with time, causing the incision site to flatten and the meridian 90 degrees away to steepen. Although the amount of flattening was by no means constant given the same size incision, the surgeon could take advantage of wound location to modify preexisting astigmatism. For example, against-the-rule astigmatism (the steep axis is horizontal) is reduced by placing the incision temporally, causing a flattening of this meridian. With these larger incisions, wound modification could be affected by the placement and location of the incision, as well as by the type of suture material used and the tension on the suture.

Astigmatism can be classified as regular or irregular (Figure 7-1). In regular astigmatism, the axis of the flat and steep meridians is 90 degrees apart. Toric spectacle correction achieves excellent best-corrected visual acuity. We are usually concerned with regular astigmatism in refractive cataract surgery. Astigmatism is also classified as with-the-rule and against-the-rule. With-the-rule astigmatism is more common in the younger population.

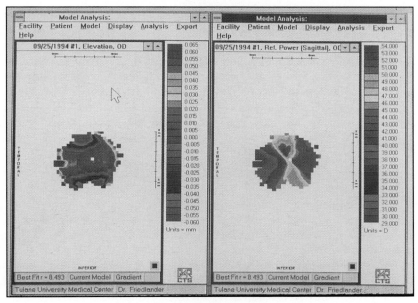

Figure 7-7. Left: non-Placido topography. PAR CT system rasterstereography. Left elevation map. The horizontal (elevated) green band corresponds to the minus cylinder. The vertical blue area (depressed) is the steeper (plus cylinder). Right: the calculated curvature map is similar to the Placido map in Figure 7-6.

Wound Size

The smaller the incision, the less the astigmatism will change postoperatively. In one study, Buzard and Shearing showed that incisions less than 5.5 mm have little or no effect on induced postoperative astigmatism.[1] With folding lenses, incisions of 3.2 mm and less are the norm. There is no question that these small incisions are preferable as far as cataract surgery is concerned; however, these small incisions prevent the surgeon from using the incision to influence either pre- or postoperative astigmatism. Larger wounds that are tied normally, especially with nylon sutures, will flatten in time. Placement of these incisions in the steeper meridian will flatten the steep meridian, thereby reducing astigmatism. If, for example, the patient has excessive with-the-rule astigmatism, a superiorly placed incision would, in time, flatten the vertical meridian and steepen the horizontal meridian. If against-the-rule astigmatism were present preoperatively, a temporal incision would, in time, flatten the steep horizontal meridian and steepen the vertical meridian.

Placement of the Incision

The closer the incision is to the cornea, the greater the effect on the astigmatism. Incisions can be divided into corneal, limbal, and scleral incisions. Corneal incisions have the advantage of no bleeding but are greatly affected by the size of the wound and tension of the sutures. Because of the avascularity of the cornea, wound healing is slow. Scleral incisions, on the other hand, are subject to bleeding, tend to heal rapidly, and have less influence on astigmatism. Limbal incisions offer the advantages of moderate avascularity and limited induced astigmatism without the drawbacks of either the scleral or corneal incisions. Both frown-shaped and straight incisions induce less astigmatism than incisions parallel to the limbus.[5,6] I classify the blue line incision (Chapter 5) as a posterior limbal incision. As such, it incorporates the best features of both corneal and scleral incisions. Astigmatism is rarely affected when the cataract extraction is combined with a foldable intraocular lens.

Suture Material

Nylon is the most flexible and easiest suture to handle. It will readily stretch and will also hydrolyze in time. Usually the younger the patient, the more rapidly the nylon dissolves. When penetrating keratoplasty is performed on older patients, 3 years are generally required for a portion of a continuous 10-0 nylon suture to dissolve. The same suture material will dissolve in 6 to 8 months in patients in their teens or early 20s. Wounds tied with nylon will loosen and flatten in time. Merselene (Ethicon, Inc, Somerville, NJ) has the least elasticity and does not hydrolyze. 10-0 Merselene is my suture of choice in astigmatism repair. Although some surgeons prefer 11-0 Merselene, I find that the 10-0 has less tendency to cheese wire.

Tension on the Sutures

Suture tension can initially modify astigmatism. At the outset, tightly tied nylon sutures steepen the radius of curvature of the adjacent cornea. Over time, the nylon stretches and finally degrades, producing the opposite effect of flattening and therefore reducing or negating the initial effect. Merselene suture is a better choice to achieve permanent wound tension. Although there is eventually some degradation of the wound, especially with larger incisions, the effect is decidedly more permanent than with nylon. Conversely, tying the sutures loosely, especially with nylon, guarantees wound slippage and flattening. This method of wound modification is inaccurate and should be avoided.

The propensity for sutureless small cataract incisions have eliminated both wound location and suture material as factors in manipulating pre-existing astigmatism. The remaining approaches to the reduction of astigmatism, whether before, during, or after cataract extraction, are limited to either incisional or laser keratotomy. At present, the role of laser keratotomy is constrained. To date, only simple and compound myopic astigmatism have been approved by the FDA. Even worse, the postsurgical reduction of astigmatism by laser is denied by Medicare and most third-party carriers. Attempts to convince the above parties have universally met with failure. It is an unacceptable reality that patients are denied the possibility of emmetropia because of such ignorance and bureaucracy. As a result, incisional keratotomy remains our main avenue of treatment.

The two most popular types of incisional keratotomy are the straight transverse (T) cut and the arcuate incision (Figures 7-8a and b, and 7-9a and b). In the T cut, the incision length is constant and the distance from the line of sight varies. The central clear zone ranges from 5 mm to 8 mm. Clear zones less than 5 mm cause glare and actually may not be

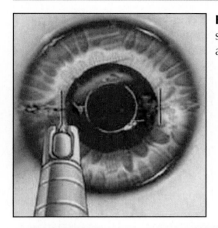

Figure 7-8a. Illustration of T cut astigmatic incisions. The incisions are horizontal, indicating an against-the-rule astigmatism.

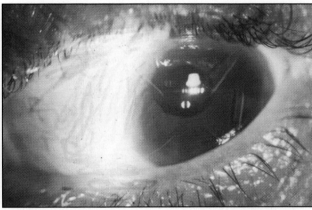

Figure 7-8b. Clinical picture of a horizontal T cut combined with a four-cut radial keratotomy.

as effective as those 5 mm or greater.[7] Given the same clear zone size and the same incision length, T cuts are about 20% to 30% less effective as arcuate incisions. As the T cut is extended to the right and left of center, the distance from the line of sight increases, thus decreasing the effect. On the contrary, in arcuate incisions, the distance from the line of sight remains the same and the length of the incision varies. Both T and arcuate cuts are age dependent and have greater efficacy with increasing years. We feel there is a practical age limit for incisional keratotomy candidates. We are most reluctant to perform astigmatic cuts on patients over 80 years old. On several occasions, such patients have lost two lines of best-corrected spectacle acuity secondary to induced irregular astigmatism. Three of these patients had paired T cuts with 8 mm clear zones.

We have included two T cut nomograms, the first is Buzard's and the second is ours (Tables 7-3 and 7-4). Note that incision length differs in the two nomograms. As little as a 0.5 mm divergence can alter the amount of astigmatism corrected. Our T cuts are always paired. For astigmatic corrections greater than 3 diopters, we no longer perform T cuts with 5 mm clear zones and instead opt for the Canrobert C procedure.

As noted above, in arcuate incisions, the distance from the visual axis is constant and the length of the incision varies. Incision length is measured in degrees. Although cadaver eye studies showed that a 7 mm clear zone may not be ideal,[8] it is the clinically preferred distance from the line of sight in arcuate incisions. Buzard's nomogram for arcuate incisions is presented in Table 7-5.

Figure 7-9a. Arcuate incisions. Given the length and same optical zone, arcuate is more effective because the arcuate is always the same distance from the visual axis.

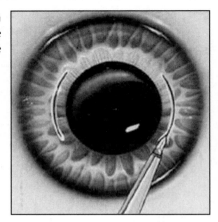

Figure 7-9b. Slit lamp picture of arcuate incisions (combined with radial keratotomy).

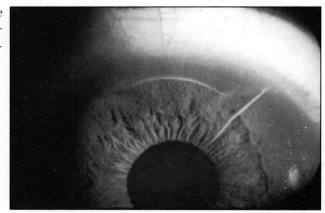

In my opinion, I find that 30-degree incisions are useless. Instead, I initially use the 45-degree or 60-degree length and reserve the 90-degree for enhancements. The 90-degree arcuate may occasionally create a disastrous overcorrection. Handling an undercorrection is far preferable to attempting to decrease an overcorrection. Although 45-degree or 60-degree incisions may not achieve the full correction initially, it is relatively simple to enhance the original surgery with a secondary procedure.

Because incisions flatten the cornea adjacent to where they are placed and 180 degrees away, the incisions are always placed in the steeper meridian. Not only will the steeper meridian flatten, but the quadrants 90 degrees away will also steepen. This is called coupling. When the coupling ratio is 1:1, the spherical equivalent will remain the same. In lower degrees of astigmatism, this transition is usually smooth and symmetrical, producing a spherical correction. In higher degrees of astigmatism, however, the area between the steep and flat meridians may not respond symmetrically. In this case, the base of the change is not spherical and instead assumes a pyramidal shape. Clinically, the best-corrected spectacle acuity will drop. This situation is avoided by using the Canrobert C procedure. The technique will be discussed later in this chapter.

Table 7-3

Buzard T-Cut Nomogram

OZ	Age										
	20	25	30	35	40	45	50	55	60	65	70
5.00	2.55	2.78	3.00	3.23	3.45	3.68	3.90	4.13	4.35	4.58	4.80
5.50	1.70	1.85	2.00	2.15	2.30	2.45	2.60	2.75	2.90	3.05	3.20
6.00	0.85	0.93	1.00	1.08	1.15	1.23	1.30	1.38	1.45	1.53	1.60
7.00	0.64	0.69	0.75	0.81	0.86	0.92	0.98	1.03	1.09	1.14	1.20

Table 7-4

*Friedlander Nomogram for Paired T Cuts**

OZ	Age											
	20	30	35	40	45	50	55	60	65	70	75	80
5.00	2.55	3.00	3.23	3.45	3.68	3.90	4.13	4.35	4.58	4.80	5.03	5.25
5.50	2.13	2.50	2.69	2.88	3.06	3.25	3.44	3.63	3.81	4.00	4.19	4.38
6.00	1.70	2.00	2.15	2.30	2.45	2.60	2.75	2.90	3.05	3.20	3.35	3.50
6.50	1.28	1.50	1.61	1.73	1.84	1.95	2.06	2.18	2.29	2.40	2.51	2.63
7.00	0.85	1.00	1.08	1.15	1.23	1.30	1.38	1.45	1.53	1.60	1.68	1.75

Blue areas represent a refractive error that is too low to correct.
*All T-cut incisions are 3 mm long.

Table 7-5

*Buzard Arcuate Incision Nomogram**

Degree of Arc	Age												
	20	25	30	35	40	45	50	55	60	65	70	75	80
45	1.70	1.85	2.00	2.15	2.30	2.45	2.60	2.75	2.90	3.05	3.20	3.35	3.50
60	2.55	2.78	3.00	2.23	3.45	3.68	3.60	4.13	4.35	4.58	4.80	5.03	5.25
90	3.40	3.70	4.00	4.30	4.60	4.90	5.20	5.50	5.80	6.10	6.40	6.70	7.00

*7-mm optical zone.

Figure 7-10. Friedlander T cut marker.

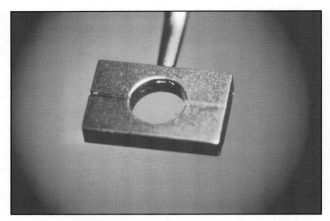

Figure 7-11. Friedlander arcuate marker.

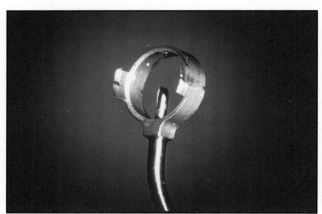

When to Address the Astigmatism and What Technique to Use

Theoretically, the astigmatic correction may be performed either before, after, or during lens extraction. We do not attempt to correct the astigmatism prior to cataract surgery. Differentiation between corneal and lenticular astigmatism is problematic at best. In theory, one should be able to differentiate between the two by comparing the keratometric and refractive astigmatism. In actuality, the presence of a cataract may distort the refraction. Even if the media is clear, there is no guarantee that the preoperative emmetropia will be maintained postoperatively.

How about performing astigmatism keratotomy at the time of cataract surgery? Although small incisions have relatively little influence on astigmatism, they have been shown to produce up to 0.50 diopters (D), resulting in flattening in the axis of the incision. Gills has advocated a popular approach to the intraoperative reduction of astigmatism: incisions are made in front of the limbus intraoperatively after IOL implantation (St. Luke's Cataract & Laser Institute pamphlet). Limbal incisions offer the advantage of reducing the irregular astigmatism and glare that are sometimes associated with incisions placed in closer proximity to the visual axis.

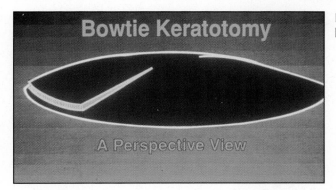

Figure 7-12. Illustration of bow tie keratotomy.

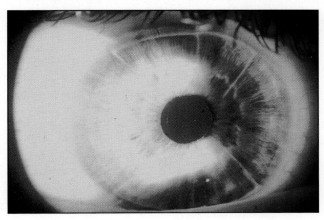

Figure 7-13. Clinical picture of bow tie keratotomy.

The concept of incisions near the limbus is not new. In the early 1980s, Steve Hollis popularized an operation named "bow tie keratotomy," which was based on a concept proposed by George Tate[9] (Figures 7-12 and 7-13). The limbal incisions are connected with four radial incisions to correct myopic astigmatism. Although the junctions of the limbus and radial incisions did not intersect, they did connect. Tate reasoned that because the incisions were connected at the limbus, they would not produce irregular astigmatism. Cadaver eye studies were followed by clinical trials on 12 eyes of eight patients. Although the sampling was too small for meaningful statistical analyses, it was shown that these incisions did reduce astigmatism.

In the Gills limbal incision, incision length ranges from 6.0 mm to 8.0 mm. They are either single or paired and are made in the steep meridian. Incision depth is standardized at 600 microns (Figure 7-14).

Published results are rare. One study by Budak, et al included 12 eyes.[10] The preoperative keratometric cylinder was 2.46 ± 0.81 and the mean reduction was 1.12 ± 0.74 D. Only three of the 12 eyes achieved full astigmatic correction. The other nine were undercorrected by approximately 25%. The obvious advantage of intraoperative astigmatic surgery is the possible elimination of a second surgery. Although glare is not a problem because the incisions are not near the visual axis, there are some disadvantages to limbal incisions: undercorrection, large incision size, and limbal bleeding.

Many surgeons, including ourselves, prefer astigmatic correction postoperatively. Do not be in a hurry to correct the astigmatism. Even with small incision surgery, the refraction may

Figure 7-14. Gills limbal incision.

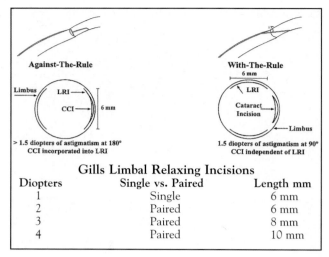

Gills Limbal Relaxing Incisions

Diopters	Single vs. Paired	Length mm
1	Single	6 mm
2	Paired	6 mm
3	Paired	8 mm
4	Paired	10 mm

continue to fluctuate for several months. Only after the refraction has stabilized will the astigmatism correction be stable and meaningful. Consider the uncorrected visual acuity for both distance and near. If the sphere and cylinder are fairly equal with opposite signs, the patient may have reasonably good distance and near vision.[11] In this example, any attempt to eliminate the astigmatism will result in poorer vision. If astigmatism of 3 D or less is to be corrected, we prefer arcuate keratotomy with a 7-mm clear zone. This procedure can be performed at the slit lamp (see Chapter 5). If a surgical microscope is preferred, we recommend the following procedure:

- Instruct the patient to sit up and opposite the surgeon.
- Anesthetize the ocular surface with proparacaine.
- Mark the cornea with a skin marking pen (coarse tip) just inside the limbus at the 12, 6, 3, and 9 o'clock positions.
- Have the patient lie down.
- Identify the center of the pupil[12] or identify the line of sight.[13]
- Next, identify and mark the steep axis.
- Mark the 7-mm clear zone and the incision length indicated on the nomogram.
- Measure the corneal thickness in that region with an ultrasonic pachymeter to determine the thinnest corneal dimension in the astigmatic quadrant.
- Set the blade at 90% or 100% of that reading.
- Mark the cornea with the appropriate arcuate marker.
- Make the incision in the uphill or Russian fashion using the vertical portion of a 10- or 15-degree trifaceted diamond blade.

As stated previously, in our hands the 30-degree length is unusable and we never use the 90-degree length initially. Of course, the excimer laser can also be used for astigmatism, but since most of the patients are covered by Medicare or have third-party policies, reimbursement is almost impossible.

For astigmatism greater than 3.50 or 4 D, I use the Canrobert C procedure. Canrobert Oliverira, an ophthalmologist from Brazil, made the following observations: normally with straight T cuts or arcuate incisions, the steep axis flattens and the flat axis steepens at a 1:1

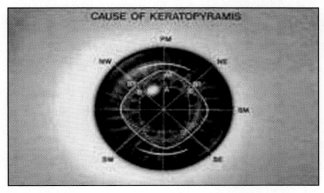

Figure 7-15. Cause of keratopyramis. With-the-rule astigmatism with incisions in the steeper meridian. The steeper meridian flattens (A to A1), but the 45-degree meridian only moves to B1 and the flat meridian does not steepen. The resulting pattern is pyramid shaped.

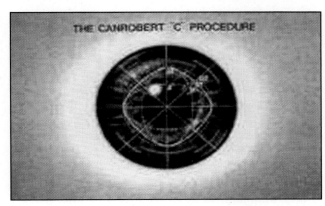

Figure 7-16. Added incisions, 45 degrees from the original, causes "rounding out" of the area between the flat and steep meridian, making the base of the original incision no longer pyramid shaped, but round.

ratio. The result in most cases, especially in lower astigmatism, is a loss of asphericity. This movement toward sphericity not only takes place in the steep and flat meridians, but in the intervening quadrants as well. When this does not occur, the base is not spherical but quadrangular. In addition, the top will be apical in shape. This resultant "keratoconoid" figure has been named keratopyramis by Oliverira (Figure 7-15). Of greater clinical significance, the patients also have a reduction in best-corrected spectacle acuity anywhere from 20/30 to 20/300. In the Canrobert C procedure, Oliverira places paired arcuate incisions in the steep meridian and also places two paired incisions at roughly 45 degrees from the original (Figure 7-16). The recommended length and distance of the incisions are listed in Table 7-6 and Figure 7-17. Coupling occurs in Canrobert C as it does in straight T cuts and arcuate incisions. When either the Canrobert C procedure or any other incisional keratotomy is used in conjunction with the excimer laser, we perform the keratotomy first and follow with LASIK within 1 month.

As with phakic refractive surgery patients, the desire of the aphakic patient for excellent visual acuity without the continuous use of spectacles or contact lenses is not only reasonable, but achievable. The ophthalmologist must take advantage of all modalities at his or her disposal to accomplish that goal.

Table 7-6

Canrobert C Procedure Nomogram for Astigmatism*
2 to 6 Diopters

Diopter	2 D	3 D	4 D	5 D	6 D**
Optical zone (mm)	7.5/8.5	7.0/8.0	6.5/7.5	6.0/7.0	6.0/7.0
Arc Length	45°/22.5°	60°/22.5°	60°/30°	60°/30°	60°/45°

*For patients less than 40 years old. For patients older than 40 years, increase the optical zone by 0.5 mm.

**Please note that on 6 D "C" incisions, the 45° incision shifts 15° toward the steep meridian.

References

1. Buzard KA, Shearing SP. Comparison of postoperative astigmatism with incisions of varying length closed with horizontal sutures and with no sutures. *J Cataract Refract Surg.* 1991;17(Suppl):734-9.

2. Duke-Elder SS, Abrams D. Dioptric imagery of the eye. In: Duke-Elder SS, ed. *System of Ophthalmology.* Vol V. St Louis, Mo: CV Mosby Co; 1970: 93-102.

3. Buzard KA, Shearing SP. Comparison of postoperative astigmatism with incisions of varying length closed with horizontal sutures and with no sutures. *J Cataract Refract Surg.* 1991;17(Suppl):734-9.

4. Holladay JT, Lynn MJ, Waring GD, Gemmill M, Keehn GC, Fielding B. The relationship of visual acuity, refractive error, and pupil size after radial keratotomy. *Arch Ophthalmol.* 1991;109(1):70-6.

5. Sinskey R, Stoppel J. Induced astigmatism in a 6.0 mm no stitch frown incision. *J Cataract Refract Surg.* 1994;20(July):406-409.

6. Singer J. Frown incision for minimizing induced astigmatism after small incision cataract surgery with rigid optic intraocular lens implantation. *J Cataract Refract Surg.* 1991;17:677-688.

7. Lavery G, Lindstrom R. Trapezoidal astigmatic keratotomy in human cadaver eyes. *J Refract Surg.* 1985;1:18-24.

8. Sabates MA, Buzard KA, Friedlander MH, Cortinas MB. Induction of astigmatism by straight transverse corneal incisions, 45 degrees long, at different clear zones in human cadaver eyes. (Published erratum appears in *J Refract Corneal Surg.* 1994;10(4):479.) *J Refract Corneal Surg.* 1994;10(3):327-32.

9. Tate GJ, Friedlander M, Goode M. *Bow Tie Keratotomy: A New Form of Astigmatic Keratotomy.* Southern Pine, NC: Caroline Eye Associates.

10. Budak K, Friedman NJ, Koch DD. Limbal relaxing incisions with cataract surgery. *J Refract Surg.* 1998;24(4):503-8.

11. Sawusch M, Guyton D. Optimal astigmatism to enhance depth of focus after cataract surgery. *Ophthalmol.* 1991;98:1027-1029.

12. Uozato H, Guyton D. Centering corneal surgical procedures. *Am J Ophthalmol.* 1987;103:264-275.

13. Buzard K. Optical aspects of refractive surgery. In: Elander R, Rich L, Robin J, eds. *Principles and Practice of Refractive Surgery.* Philadelphia, Pa: WB Sanders Company; 1997: 39-74.

(in the range of 1 to 2 D) and suffer from both hyperopia and presbyopia. The classification and treatment of hyperopia should therefore reflect the basic epidemiology of hyperopic patients. We therefore define low hyperopia as 0 to 2 D, moderate hyperopia from 2 to 6 D, and high hyperopia above 6 D. In addition, we qualify the use of lens exchange on two basic principles: over age 50 and/or hyperopia greater than 2 D, above which we believe the results of corneal hyperopic refractive surgery are less satisfactory at this time. Hyperopia is relatively uncommon until the age of 50, at which time there is a marked increase in hyperopia. The incidence of hyperopia is much more common at ages 65 to 74 (67%) than it is at 43 to 54 (22%).[4]

The purpose of this chapter is to propose clear lens extraction with IOL implantation as the primary means of correcting hyperopia, high myopia, and in all patients other than those with accommodation (and even in patients with accommodation) if hyperopia is greater than 2 to 3 D. Previous articles have demonstrated both the good results associated with clear lens extraction[5,6] with small numbers and the relatively poor results obtained with hexagonal keratotomy,[7,8,9,10,11,12,13] epikeratophakia,[14,15,16,17,18] hyperopic ALK,[19] thermokeratoplasty,[20,21,22,23] and even hyperopic photorefractive keratectomy (PRK) and laser-assisted in situ keratomileusis (LASIK).[24,25,26]

While hyperopic PRK and LASIK have promise for producing better results than the others, particularly with adjustments to the ablation profile, it remains true that most of these patients are in their mid to late 50s with at least mild lens changes which, in our opinion, substantially alter the appropriate mode of action. Even if corneal operations were markedly successful for hyperopia, the onset of lens changes means that refractive errors will change and even the application of PRK may well promote the onset of further lens changes. We believe these important issues have not been properly addressed in previous studies when considering the correction of hyperopia. In the instance of a patient 30 to 40 years old with myopia or mild hyperopia, a reasonable expectation of 10 to 20 years of benefit can be expected; whereas in a patient in his or her late 50s with early lens changes, a corneal operation is unlikely to provide benefit for more than 5 to 10 years. In distinction, a clear lens extraction with IOL implantation can provide a correction with the same duration as the myopic operation—at least 10 to 20 years. All of these point to the need to consider the patient over age 50 in a separate category and to consider lens extraction as a primary modality.

Risk

Every surgical procedure has risk, and lens exchange is no exception. The primary areas of risk are retinal detachment, endophthalmitis, expulsive hemorrhage, vitreous loss/torn capsule/retained nuclear fragments, endothelial damage and/or wound incompetence. Using the transconjunctival blue line incision,[27] wound incompetence is virtually unknown. In approximately 5000 cases using this incision we have never had a wound leak, and historically, the scleral tunnel incision has been shown to be a remarkably stable and strong incision, particularly if it is kept within the "incisional funnel."[28,29] Endophthalmitis has been reported as a problem with the clear corneal incision,[30] and the wound construction can be relatively easily compromised, resulting in wound leakage and a setup for endophthalmitis. We believe this is a strong incentive to consider the blue line incision, in addition to the relative astigmatic neutrality of this wound construction. Any intraocular surgery is associated with some endothelial cell loss and, of course, IOLs placed in the anterior chamber are more likely to encounter this problem.[31,32]

Werblin studied the issue of long-term endothelial stability after IOL implantation in several models using different types of intraocular lenses.[33] He found that posterior chamber IOL implantation after phacoemulsification was associated with about a 10% cell loss that was stable after 3 years in patients followed up to 6 years. Problems with rupture of the capsule and/or vitreous loss should be rare in relatively young patients with soft nuclei, but it is important to note that technique-related issues should be resolved before entering into lens exchange surgery. With good technique, related problems such as CME should be rare.[34] Similarly, with larger incisions that were not self-sealing and with older patients, expulsive hemorrhage was a more significant complication. This complication is rare in younger patients and with a small self-sealing incision, it should be easy to raise IOP and inhibit progression of this problem.

The area of greatest concern is the problem of retinal detachment associated with lens extraction. The concerns revolve primarily around patients with myopia since retinal detachment rates are much lower in patients with hyperopia and the results have been relatively good.[35,36,37] Few results are available for clear lens exchange in myopia, so most studies examine the rates of retinal detachment in cataract patients. By their nature, these patients are usually older with more difficult surgery, and the rates should only be taken as a general measure of the actual rate. Also, the most common studies involve the rate of retinal detachment with older surgical techniques with larger wounds and without capsulorrhexis with rates of 1.3% to 6% per year for extracapsular cataract extraction (ECCE) surgeries.[38,39] In patients with high myopia (>10 D), the natural rate of retinal detachment is approximately 0.7% per year,[40] so the rate of retinal detachment is increased with ECCE surgeries and particularly after YAG laser capsulotomy. We believe that it is important to maintain the lens-iris diaphragm to minimize the movement of vitreous, and without a capsulotomy, the barrier is incomplete. We create a capsulotomy smaller than the IOL optic (usually about 5 mm, and when YAG laser is performed, the opening is made through an undilated pupil [approximately 4 mm]). This ensures a tight lens-iris diaphragm and minimal movement of vitreous. Verzella performed one of the earliest and largest studies of lens exchange in high myopia and reported a retinal detachment rate of only 0.7%,[41,42] approximately the same as the rate without lens surgery. Unfortunately, the visual results were less than impressive, with 89% within 6 D of the intended correction due in large part to a limited range of available IOL powers. While Verzella required preoperative and yearly retinal checks, other authors have insisted on prophylactic retinal treatments, apparently with relatively good results. Colin[43] studied 49 eyes of 28 patients with approximately two-thirds treated with retinal photocoagulation prior to surgery. With a 4-year follow-up, the incidence of retinal detachment was 1.9%, and the incidence of YAG capsulotomy was 36.7%. Uncorrected visual acuity of 20/40 or better was achieved in 38% of patients. Eighty-two percent treated with YAG laser had 20/100 or better versus 62% of untreated eyes. The increased rate of retinal detachment, which Colin has recently reported to be even higher, might be explained by the fact that some of the patients underwent ECCE and/or the failure of prophylactic photocoagulation. Centurion[44] has also reported on patients treated with prophylactic photocoagulation and followed for 6 years. In 35 patients, no retinal detachments were noted, although the visual results were again a little disappointing, with only 75% of the patients with 2 D or less of residual myopia.

We have two prospective studies examining the issue of retinal detachment. In the first series, 402 eyes undergoing clear lens exchange have been followed for 3 years. Of these eyes,

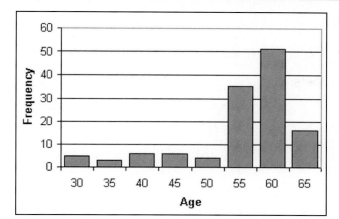

Figure 8-1. Age distribution of 126 patients prior to myopic clear lens exchange.

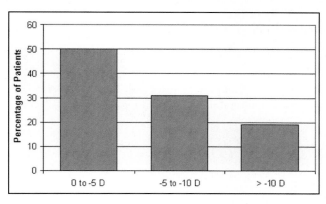

Figure 8-2. Distribution of preoperative spherical equivalent for 126 patients prior to myopic clear lens exchange.

126 were myopic with an age distribution shown in Figure 8-1, which shows the majority of the patients older than 50 years. In all myopic patients, a preoperative retinal exam was performed prior to surgery. In Figure 8-2 we see the distribution of myopia with the majority of patients who have a low degree of myopia. Of these 402 eyes, we had one retinal detachment, as shown in Table 8-1, 1 month after YAG laser capsulotomy for a retinal detachment rate of 0.25% for the entire series of clear lens exchange or 0.8% for the myopic eyes. Of interest is the final uncorrected vision of 20/25, which shows little visual compromise from the detachment and the fact that this patient was a moderate myope with a preoperative spherical equivalent of -5.50 D. A second series of 2800 eyes undergoing cataract surgery with the blue line incision and phacoemulsification were followed for 3 years. In this group, three patients had a retinal detachment, all myopic as shown in Table 8-1 for a retinal detachment rate of 0.1%. Surprisingly, the final visual acuities were all better than 20/40 and not all patients underwent YAG laser capsulotomy. Some authors have suggested an increased incidence of retinal detachment among women, although this data shows no such tendency. Colon's recent data suggests an increased tendency for retinal detachment after 4 to 6 years. Several issues bring this finding into question. First, not all cases were performed with a small incision phacoemulsification—some of the cases were performed with ECCE. Second, the YAG laser technique is not defined and the lens/iris diaphragm may have been compromised, resulting in a higher incidence of retinal detachment. Finally, the incidence of retinal detachment in a small series more than 5 years after the original lens surgery makes

Table 8-1

Retinal Detachment After Clear Lens and Cataract Surgery

Type of surgery	Clear lens exchange	CE\IOL	CE\IOL	CE\IOL
Age	59	54	66	57
Sex	Male	Male	Male	Male
Preop axial length	25.97 mm	26.98 mm	27.03 mm	25.89
Time to RD after surgery	4 months	9 months	1 year	2 years
YAG	Yes	Yes	No	No
Final VAOC	20/20	20/30	20/25*	20/30

*Reading vision

CE = cataract extraction; RD = retinal detachment; VAOC = visual acuity without correction

the issue of cause and effect tenuous. Each year that passes carries additional factors into the equation that must be considered before assigning the blame to a long past event.

Surgical Technique

The surgical technique is essentially the same as cataract surgery, but some important points need to be made. Much of the discussion with lens exchange revolves around complications, although the actual technique is extremely important not only in regard to the initial procedure but also in regard to "enhancement procedures." We believe that it is important to maintain ocular pressure during the procedure, and failure to do so may result in higher rates of retinal detachment. Additionally, as discussed earlier, we use a 5-mm capsulorrhexis and a small YAG laser capsulotomy when required. Clearly, any complication is magnified in a cosmetic application and with this in mind, the surgeon should carefully evaluate each aspect of the procedure, particularly as it relates to complication and infection. We believe this is particularly true as it relates to the choice of incision, and while the clear corneal incision can be performed without complication in the majority of patients, we believe it is relatively unforgiving and more likely to leak and possibly allow an infection than a scleral tunnel incision.

We also believe that the surgeon should review his or her results with respect to refractive outcome. If uncorrected vision is not better than 20/40 in the majority of patients, a possible review of both preoperative workup and surgical technique may be appropriate before making the move to refractive lens exchange. Additionally, any refractive procedure requires the ability to enhance the result, and the surgeon should consider whether his or her ability to enhance both astigmatic and spherical results after the original surgery are adequate and, equally important, cost effective. LASIK may be used to correct both astigmatic and spherical errors, but in most cases will not be a cost-effective procedure unless utilized in small numbers. Additionally, LASIK in the older patient, in our experience, is often complicated by epithelial disruption, which can result in some cases in prolonged visual recovery. The three basic techniques that form the basics of "lens exchange" in our practice are the basic lens removal technique, 3-mm sutureless IOL exchange technique, and the technique for slit lamp astigmatic incisions, which are all described in this book.

Basic Lens Removal Technique

There are as many ways to remove a lens as there are surgeons, but in very general terms we use the blue line cataract incision (a transconjunctival incision created with a diamond blade), and we do not believe in the use of limbal relaxing incisions at the time of cataract surgery because of the limited effect and possible long-term instability. This technique is described in more detail in a recent publication.[27]

We usually perform the blue line incision superiorly, although it may be applied in any meridian. We utilize a trapezoid diamond knife (Buzard Blue Line Knife, Mastel Precision). The diamond has a 2.7 mm inside and a 3.0 mm outside width and is 6 mm long with a truncated tip 100 microns in length to provide better control during creation of the incision. Of particular interest, the blade is at least 2 mm longer than the standard cataract diamond knife, allowing for the more posterior placement of the external wound and a generally longer tunnel incision.

The eye is stabilized by grasping in the inferior conjunctiva and drawing the eye downward with a .5 forceps. The blue line incision is constructed by first creating a 4-mm incision through the conjunctiva about 1.5 to 2 mm behind the surgical limbus with the side of the diamond knife (represented by an anatomic appearance of a blue line). In the usual case, the conjunctiva will naturally sag away from the incision and the resulting conjunctival gaping will create a "mini-peritomy." While bleeding is not a significant problem, the assistant applies steady drops to maintain visualization of the exterior incision. The knife is placed parallel to the posterior sclera, and pressure is applied to slightly indent the sclera with the knife pushing forward to begin the scleral tunnel incision. As the incision evolves, progressive pressure is placed on the heel of the diamond knife to prevent early interior entry caused by the changing curvature at the limbus between the sclera and cornea. Finally, when the tip of the knife approaches the desired location for the internal corneal incision, the heel of the knife is rotated slightly upward, creating a slight dimple in the corneal surface. The corneal dimple is relieved when the tip of the knife penetrates Descemet's membrane. The knife is then inserted until the "shoulders" are at the level of the internal corneal incision, which is 2.7 mm in width.

The blue line incision described above results in an approximately square 3 x 3 mm scleral tunnel incision. Light cautery is then applied to the conjunctival edge to control bleeding. A side-port incision is made with the same diamond knife, viscoelastic is instilled in the anterior chamber, and the capsulorrhexis is performed with a cystotome. Hydrodissection and hydrodelineation are performed and a derivation of the standard divide and conquer technique phacoemulsification is used to remove the soft lens. At present, we like the STAAR three-piece silicone IOL with a 6.30 optic and a 13.50 overall diameter implantation (STAAR AQ2010V). We like this lens because it goes into a very small incision and is easy to remove with the IOL exchange technique we will discuss later in this book. Viscoelastic material is removed with irrigation and aspiration. A wound leakage test is performed by injecting saline through the side port, checking along the incision and on the

Figure 8-3. Age distribution of 68 eyes in 34 patients prior to clear lens exchange.

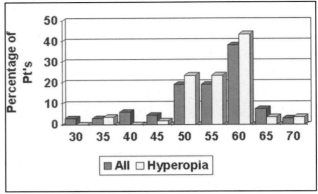

Figure 8-4. Preoperative distribution of spherical equivalent for hyperopic patients.

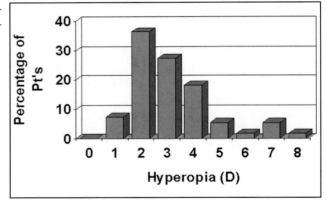

sclera. Of interest is the fact that hydration of the cornea, which is frequently required to obtain a watertight wound in the clear-corneal incision (about 20% in our experience), is rarely required with the blue line incision (about 5%).

Small Clinical Study

We performed clear lens exchange on 68 eyes of 34 patients ranging in age from 30 to 67 years old (average 52 + 9 years) (Figure 8-3). Of these, 13 patients were male and 21 were female. Twenty-five eyes received a monovision correction, while 43 were corrected for distance. Surgery was performed on an outpatient basis using either a sutureless incision (57 eyes) or a single horizontal suture (11 eyes) in patients in whom a foldable lens could not be obtained to meet the power requirements of the case.

Mean best-corrected vision prior to surgery was 20/20, while mean preoperative uncorrected vision was 20/100. Mean preoperative spherical equivalent for hyperopic patients was +2.72 + 1.59 D (Figure 8-4), and mean spherical equivalent for the myopic patients was -12.30 + 7.94 D (Figure 8-5). Mean keratometry was 43.65 + 2.13, and average cell count was 2700 cells\mm^2 prior to surgery.

Preoperatively, the same general routine used for our cataract patients was followed. All eyes were examined for systemic problems. Ocular examination included corrected and

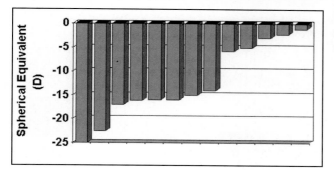

Figure 8-5. Preoperative spherical equivalent of myopic patients.

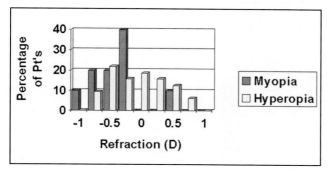

Figure 8-6. Postoperative distribution of spherical equivalent for myopic and hyperopic patients.

uncorrected distance visual acuity, manifest refraction, keratometry (Zeiss Humphrey, Dublin, Calif), corneal topography (EyeSys, Sacramento), cell count (Konan, Mumbal, India), and axial length (Nidek, Gamagori, Japan). Calculations were done using the Hoffer IOL calculation computer program (Hoffer, Santa Monica, Calif) aiming for a postoperative spherical equivalent value of -0.50 for distance and a "monovision" system dependent on patient desires and testing prior to surgery, usually aiming for a postoperative result of -1.50 to -2.00 D for reading.

Results

No significant operative or postoperative complications occurred, notably no retinal complications occurred. The average postoperative spherical equivalent was -0.11 + 0.43 D for the distance eyes (Figure 8-6) and -1.79 + 0.53 D for the monovision eyes (Figure 8-7). The near correction corresponds closely to the intended goal of -1.5 to -1.75 D correction in the reading eye of monovision. The refraction results from 6 weeks onward did not differ; refractions seemed relatively stable after that point. The mean uncorrected visual acuity improved from 20/100 preoperatively to an average of 20/30 with no lines lost on BCVA (best-corrected visual acuity) (Figure 8-8). The 20/30 uncorrected vision figure includes some patients in whom best-corrected vision is less than 20/20 due to refractive amblyopia. The average percentage of endothelial cell loss measured at the 6 month visit was 9.8 + 2.1%. Average preoperative astigmatism was 0.94 D (range 2.88 D to 0.25 D) for patients with near corrections and 1.27 D (range 4.38 D to 0.00 D) for patients with distance correction. Astigmatic relaxing incisions were performed in 25 eyes with reduction of postoperative astigmatism to under 1 D in all patients. All patients seemed satisfied with the sur-

Figure 8-7. Postoperative distribution of spherical equivalent for reading eyes of monovision patients.

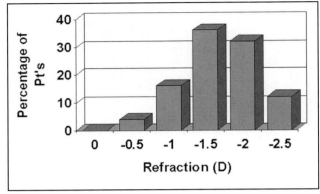

Figure 8-8. Postoperative distribution of uncorrected visual acuity.

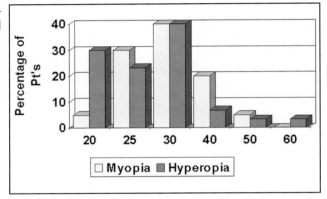

gery. In particular, the patients were happy with the monovision corrections, which we believe is heavily dependent on careful preoperative discussion and assessment of success with monovision by means of contact lens trials and education.

Enhancement operations were necessary in a total of 17 patients, in addition to the aforementioned 25 patients treated at the slit lamp with relaxing incisions for astigmatism. One patient was treated with LASIK for mild unexpected myopia and one patient was treated with LASIK to reverse a monovision correction. Three-millimeter sutureless IOL exchange was necessary in three patients due to residual hyperopia. No complications were encountered with any of these enhancements.

Discussion

The concept of clear lens extraction with IOL implantation is not new and has been previously proposed by other authors.[45,46] What has not changed are the relatively poor results obtained with corneal manipulation for hyperopia, even with newer techniques of thermokeratoplasty, hyperopic PRK, and hyperopic LASIK. For small amounts of hyperopic correction (under 2 to 4 D), these corneal techniques can be successful with minimal loss of best-corrected visual acuity and few complications. However, for larger degrees of hyperopia there seems to be a common problem experienced by virtually all corneal hyperopic procedures, which is loss of best-corrected visual acuity with even very mild decentrations of the procedure. Why the cornea tolerates relatively large decentrations for myopic procedures and yet even a small decentration of hyperopic or steepening procedures causes loss of BCVA is somewhat of a mystery. In addition, many, if not most, of the patients presenting for hyperopic corrections are in the age group of 50 and above; in fact, as seen from our data, most are in their mid to late 50s. As patients enter into their middle and late 50s, lens changes begin to occur that cannot be classified as cataracts, but under conditions of bright or poor lighting can result in a loss of detail, which may be noticeable to the patient following a corneal refractive procedure. We have observed several patients with such lens changes that underwent myopic and hyperopic LASIK procedures with resulting best-corrected vision of 20/25 to 20/30 and significant complaints of poor vision with increased glare following the procedure. Observation at the slit lamp reveals small increases in nuclear sclerosis and often the development of subtle anterior and posterior subcapsular changes. Removal of the lenses and substitution with IOLs resolved the complaints in all of these patients and resulted in best-corrected visions of 20/20 in most of these cases. For this reason, and because we believe that even mild lenticular changes can result in refractive changes that can alter the refractive effect of corneal surgery, we now carefully evaluate even mild lenticular changes in patients 50 years and older for both myopic and hyperopic surgeries. If sufficient changes are present, as evidenced by slit lamp observation and/or glare, lens surgery is chosen to correct the refractive error rather than laser corneal surgery. In fact, lens refractive surgery has become the surgery of choice for patients over age 50, and LASIK is restricted to special cases.

As a final inducement to consider lens replacement as a preferred treatment for hyperopia and in general for patients over age 50, we note the markedly improved surgical techniques now available for cataract surgery. The small incision lens extraction with capsulorrhexis is much safer due to the self-sealing nature of the incision and maintenance of the anterior chamber during even violent patient movement and/or coughing. In-the-bag placement with the capsulorrhexis provides a superior fixation of the intraocular lens with subsequent improvement of refractive results, which have already been improved by better calculation formulas prior to surgery. In fact, the utilization of lens replacement surgery is really a reflection of our changing attitudes toward cataract surgery as a whole. Today, it is our goal to provide every cataract patient with an uncorrected postoperative visual acuity of 20/40 or better, and we reach this goal in our general population of cataract patients in more than 90% of the cases, often on the first day after surgery. This attitude is not unique to us, but in fact has become a common goal in many, if not most, of the cataract practices in the United States. If the "value added" refractive results that can be obtained with small incision sutureless cataract surgery and relatively minor astigmatic corrections are made available to patients with cataracts, why then should they be denied to younger patients? The only subset of patients who might give a second thought to lens corrective surgery would be patients with active accommodation younger than age 38 to 40.

However, in our experience, patients with severe degrees of hyperopia (greater than 2 to 3 D) are more than willing to give up accommodation for better uncorrected vision, as evidenced by a 32-year-old patient included in our study with 6 D of hyperopia preoperatively and 20/25 to 20/30 vision postoperatively. This patient is absolutely thrilled with the results of his surgery and feels the loss of accommodation was a minor price to pay for the resolution of his hyperopia. While all younger patients may not have the same response, it is certainly present in some; and for those who desire an alternative, this relatively small group of patients might benefit from the phakic ICL (intraocular contact lens).

Myopic patients have the additional consideration of retinal detachment, yet this complication seems markedly decreased with more recent techniques and may even be reduced if appropriate retinal consultation is obtained. Even if retinal detachment occurs, modern retinal reattachment can be very successful. If the retinal detachment occurs years after the surgery, it is not entirely clear that the detachment is related to the lens exchange surgery.

In summary, clear lens extraction is a safe and predictable means to correct refractive errors of virtually any degree. The recent advances in wound construction and cataract removal have made clear lens extraction a natural outgrowth of the trend toward refractive phacoemulsification occurring in cataract surgery as a whole. Finally, the issue of early lenticular changes in patients over age 50 with the possibility of progression of these lenticular deficits with the application of the excimer laser makes clear lens extraction a superior approach for this particular group.

References

1.   Bullimore MA, Gilmartin B. Hyperopia and presbyopia: etiology and epidemiology. In: Sher, ed. *Surgery for Hyperopia and Presbyopia*. Baltimore, Md: Williams & Wilkins; 1987: 3-10.

2.   van Alphern GWHM. On emmetropia and ametropia. *Ophthalmologica Supplementum*. 1961;142:1-92.

3.   Sorsby A, Benjamin B, Davey, JB, et al. *Emmetropia and its Aberrations*. London: Her Majesty's Stationery Office; 1957: 293.

4.   Wang Q, Klein BEK, Klein R, et al. Refractive status in the Beaver Dam Eye Study. *Invest Ophthalmol Vis Sci*. 1994;35:4344-4347.

5.   Isfahani AH, Salz J. Clear lens extraction with intraocular lens implantation for the correction of hyperopia. In: Sher, ed. *Surgery for Hyperopia and Presbyopia*. Baltimore, Md: Williams & Wilkins: 1987;175-181.

6.   Buzard KA, Fundingsland BR. Clear lens extraction for hyperopia operative techniques in cataract and refractive surgery. <journal title> 1999;2(1):35-40.

7.   Werblin TP. Hexagonal keratotomy—should we still be trying. *J Refract Surg*. 1996;12:613-620.

8.   Grandon SC, Sanders DR, Anello RD, et al. Clinical evaluation of hexagonal keratotomy for the treatment of primary hyperopia. *J Cataract Refract Surg*. 1995;21:140-149.

9.   Grady FJ. Hexagonal keratotomy for corneal steepening. *Ophthalmic Surg*. 1988;19:622-623.

10. Basuk WL, Zisman M, Waring GO, et al. Complications of hexagonal keratotomy. *Am J Ophthalmol*. 1994;117:37-49.

11. Mendez A. Hexagonal keratotomy for hyperopia. *Proceedings of the Keratorefractive Society*. New Orleans, La; 1986.

12. Jensen RP. Hexagonal keratotomy: clinical experience with 483 eyes. *Int Ophthalmol Clin*. 1991;31:69-73.

13. Neumann AC, McCarty GR. Hexagonal keratotomy for correction of low hyperopia: preliminary results of a prospective study. *J Cataract Refract Surg*. 1988;14:265-269.

14. American Academy of Ophthalmology. Ophthalmic procedures assessment, keratophakia and keratomileusis: safety and effectiveness. *Ophthalmology*. 1992;99(8):1332-1341.

15. Ehrlich MI, Nordan LT. Epikeratophakia for the treatment of hyperopia. *J Cataract Refract Surg*. 1989;15:661-666.

16. McDonald MB, Kaufman HE, Aquavella JV, et al. The nationwide study of epikeratophakia for aphakia in adults. *Am J Ophthalmol*. 1987;103:358-365.

17. Arffa RC, Marelli TL, Morgan KS. Long-term follow-up refractive and keratometric results of pediatric epikeratophakia. *Arch Ophthmol*. 1986;104:668-670.

18. Dingeldein SA, McDonald MB. Epikeratophakia. *Int Ophthalmol Clin*. 1988;28:134-144.

19. Manche EE, Judge A, Maloney RK. Lamellar keratoplasty for hyperopia. *J Refract Surg*. 1996;12:42-49.

20. Neumann AC, Fydorov S, Sander DR. Radial thermokeratoplasty for the correction of hyperopia. *Refract Corneal Surg*. 1990;6:404-412.

21. Fydorov SN, Ivashina AI, Aleksandrova OG, Bessarabov AN. Surgical correction of compound hypermetropic and mixed astigmatism by sectoral thermal keratocoagulation. *Implants in Ophthalmology*. 1990;2:43-48.

22. Neumann AC, Sanders D, Raanan M, DeLuca M. Hyperopic thermokeratoplasty: clinical evaluation. *J Cataract Refract Surg*. 1991;17:830-838.

23. Feldman ST, Ellis W, Frucht-Pery J, Chayet A, Brown SI. Regression of effect following radial thermokeratoplasty in humans. *Refract Corneal Surg*. 1989;5:288-291.

24. Dausch D, Klein R, Schroder E. Excimer laser photorefractive keratectomy for hyperopia. *J Refract Corneal Surg*. 1993;9:20-28.

25. Dausch D, Klein R, Landesz M, Schroder E. Photorefractive keratectomy to correct astigmatism with myopia of hyperopia. *J Cataract Refract Surg*. 1994;20(suppl):252-257.

26. Buzard KA, Fundingsland BR. Excimer laser assisted in-situ keratomileusis for hyperopia. *J Cataract Ref Surg*. Submitted.

27. Buzard KA, Febbraro JL. Transconjunctival incision blue line.

28. Kohenen T, Koch DD. Methods to control astigmatism in cataract surgery. *Curr Opin Ophthalmol*. 1996;7:75-80.

29. Samuleson SW, Koch DD, Kuglen CC. Determination of maximal incision length for true small-incision surgery. *Ophthalmic Surg*. 1991;22:204-7.

30. Personal communication, Maurice John.

31. Baikoff G, Colin J. Intraocular lenses in phakic patients. *Ophthalmol Clin North Am*. 1992;4:789-795.

32. Saragoussi JJ, Cotinat F, Renard M, et al. Damage to the corneal endothelium by minus power anterior chamber intraocular lenses. *Refract Corneal Surg*. 1991;7:282-285.

33. Werblin TP. The long-term endothelial cell loss following phacoemulsification surgery: the model for evaluating endothelial damage following intraocular surgery. *Refract Corneal Surg*. 1993;9:29-35.

34. Clayman HM. Intraocular lenses. In: Duane TD, ed. *Clinical Ophthalmology*. Vol 6. New York, NY: Harper & Row; 1992; 1-33.

35. Buzard KA, Fundingsland FB. Clear lens exchange for hyperopia. *Operative Techniques in Cataract and Refractive Surgery*. 1999;1(1):35-40.

36. Lyle WA, Jin CJC. Clear lens extraction for the correction of high refractive error. *J Cataract Refract Surg*. 1994;20:273-276.

37. Siganos SD, Siganos CS, Pallikaris IG. Clear lens extraction and intraocular lens implantation in normally sighted hyperopic eyes. *J Refract Corneal Surg*. 1994;10:117-121.

38. Lindstrom RL. Retinal detachment in axial myopia. *Dev Ophthalmol*. 1987:14;37-41.

39. Praeger DL. Five year's follow-up in the surgical management of cataracts in high myopia treated with the Kelman phacoemulsification technique. *Ophthalmology*. 1979;86:2024-2033.

40. Goldberg MF. Clear lens extraction for axial myopia: an appraisal. *Ophthalmology*. 1987;94:571-598.

41. Verzella F. Microsurgery of the lens in high myopia for optical purposes. *Cataract*. 1984;1:8-12.

42. Verzella F. High myopia: refractive lensectomy and posterior chamber implants. *Cataract.* 1985;2:25-27.

43. Colin J, Robinet A. Clear lensectomy and implantation of low-power posterior chamber lens for the correction of high myopia. *Ophthalmology.* 1994:101:107-112.

44. Centurion V, Caballero JC, Medeiros OA, et al. Clear lens extraction and high myopia. *J Refract Corneal Surg.* Submitted.

45. Isfahani AH, Salz J. Clear lens extraction with intraocular lens implantation for the correction of hyperopia. In: Shear, ed. *Surgery for Hyperopia and Presbyopia.* Baltimore, Md: Williams & Wilkins; 1997; 175-181.

46. Siganos DS, Siganos CS, Pallikaris IG. Clear lens extraction and intraocular lens implantation in normally sighted hyperopic eyes. *J Refract Corneal Surg.* 1994:10:117-124.

fected by pupil size and lens decentration. Lens decentration may occur following implantation of any type of IOL—diffractive or refractive.

The diffractive optic of this MIOL directed transmitted light to two primary focal points. Fourty percent of light was devoted to distance vision, 40% to near, and 20% of light transmission was lost to higher orders of diffraction. Incoming light could be incident on any portion of the zones within the pupil and still produce two points of focus. For this reason, the diffractive lens could tolerate moderate amounts of decentration and variation in pupil size.[12] All zones of the lens surface contributed to the dual power function, unlike a Fresnel lens of distinct refractive regions. In fact, according to Simpson, there are generally distinct differences between a Fresnel lens, which is a refractive optic, and the diffractive surface of the 3M MIOL.[13]

Lindstrom reported near vision results at 1-year postoperative implantation of the diffractive MIOL compared to monofocal IOLs. With distance correction only, eyes achieving J1-J3 near acuity were found in 92% with MIOLs compared to 37% with monofocal IOLs, and 59% of bilaterally implanted 3M diffractive MIOL patients never needed spectacles. There were no statistically significant differences in corrected distance or near visual acuity when compared among eyes with pupil sizes ranging from 2.0 mm to 7.0 mm.[14]

Gimbel reported on 149 patients with bilateral 3M diffractive multifocal IOLs, finding 63% of patients needed no spectacle correction compared to 4% of monofocal cases. Multifocal patients reported significantly more visual side effects, such as glare and halos, and a greater decrease in contrast sensitivity at low contrast levels was detected among multifocal cases.[15]

A German study demonstrated a surprisingly high loss of contrast sensitivity for both 3M diffractive multifocal patients and monofocal patients. Seventy percent of MIOL patients and 56% of monofocal patients failed to meet the minimum requirements for a driver's license in Germany.[16]

Restoration of near vision with this MIOL began to be called "pseudoaccommodation" and, as expected, patient satisfaction was highest when the distance refraction was near emmetropia and astigmatism was minimal. Low hyperopic patients were found to have less problems than low myopes.[17]

An FDA advisory panel recommended approval of the diffractive MIOL in 1992 if certain strict clinical evaluations of this lens were found satisfactory, such as visual performance under various driving conditions. This MIOL was purchased by Alcon Laboratories (Fort Worth, Tex) and named the RëStor lens. Recently, Alcon has been redesigning the diffractive optic to reduce the possibility of unwanted visual imagery and is considering adding this diffractive component to the popular AcrySof acrylic IOL. Other companies, such as Pharmacia (Monrovia, Calif), have been manufacturing diffractive MIOLs. The Pharmacia Ceeon 811E lens has been extensively implanted outside of the United States.

Three-Zone Refractive MIOL

Concurrent with diffractive MIOL investigation, many other refractive designs were being studied. A variety of three-zone MIOLs, providing distance and near vision by using a near annulus at various distances from the central distance component, were manufactured by Alcon, Pharmacia, and Storz. The Storz True Vista has gained popularity, especially in European countries.

A multicenter European study reported by Knorz demonstrated excellent distance acuity

(20/40 or better in 97%) with the True Vista, except at low contrast. Near acuity was satisfactory in 64%. Dr. Knorz found that this MIOL "emphasizes the far focus."[18,19] Shoji also evaluated the True Vista MIOL and found better near acuities with the P359-TUV model, reporting 79% who obtained J1 or better near vision with distance correction only. He found that there was no significant difference in contrast sensitivity between multifocal and monofocal patients if the multifocal patients had bilateral MIOLs.[20]

Normal pupil patients can enjoy both near and distance vision, but smaller pupils can obstruct the near component with some three-zone MIOLs. However, smaller pupils may enhance contrast sensitivity. A study by Knorz and Koch demonstrated a loss of best-corrected contrast acuity with increasing pupillary size that was statistically greater with the True Vista MIOL eyes than with monofocal eyes.[21] One advantage of this lens design is that even though there is pupil dependency, distance vision is always preserved despite the loss of near acuity due to miosis.

The Array MIOL

The Allergan (Irvine, Calif) Array multifocal IOL was the first MIOL to be granted premarket approval by the FDA, receiving this status in September 1997. Over 100,000 Array MIOLs have been implanted, making the Array the most popular multifocal worldwide.

The optical composition of the Array has been termed "zonal progressive," a refractive design that incorporates five blended aspheric zones of power on the anterior surface of the optic. The central 2.1 mm of the optic is dedicated to distance vision, with the first near ring positioned from 2.1 mm to 3.4 mm followed by a distance zone, then another near zone (Figure 9-1). The Array is considered a "distance dominant" MIOL with 50% of light transmission assigned to distance vision, 13% to intermediate, and 37% to near. With the current add power of 3.5 D (2.6 D effective power at the spectacle plane), near vision of at least J3 is commonly seen, sometimes calling for an additional spectacle add with certain near vision requirements, such as very fine print. Like three-zone refractive MIOLs, the Array tends to lose a portion of its near function as the pupil becomes smaller than 2.0 mm.

The Array is currently only manufactured with a 6.0 mm silicone optic. (Plans are being made for an acrylic Array, a modification of the Sensar monofocal IOL from Allergan.) The ability to insert the foldable silicone Array through a small incision has been a real asset for this lens. Whether using folding forceps or the Allergan insertion device, the Unfolder, unwanted induced astigmatism is less likely to occur compared to rigid PMMA MIOLs.

During clinical trials before premarket approval, a number of new study methods were undertaken in order to demonstrate the relative benefits of the Array compared to monofocal IOLs. Traditionally, visual data and complication rates have been the major criteria for clinical evaluation of multifocal (and monofocal) IOLs. Array investigators employed a new concept, that of "quality of life" studying, to learn just how the multifocal vision that patients experience after Array implantation impacts their daily lives. Instead of just measuring visual acuity, quality of life assessment was used to measure visual function. In a multicenter, retrospective randomized clinical trial, the Array patients reported substantially higher quality of life ratings compared to monofocal controls, as reported by Javitt, et al.[22]

Steinert led an earlier randomized, double masked, multicenter trial to clinically evaluate the PMMA forerunner to the silicone Array, the Array MPC-25NB. The Array-implanted eyes, as expected, were found to have some loss of low contrast acuity. Glare and light sensitivity ratings were similar between Array and monofocal controls. The cumulative patient survey results showed significantly greater patient satisfaction in the Array group.[23]

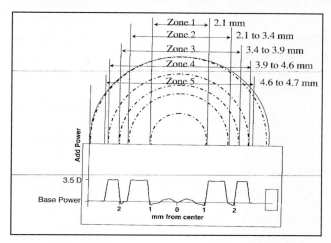

Figure 9-1. Optical composition of the Array multifocal IOL.

A more recent multicenter investigation carried out by a double-masked prospective method yielded similar clinical results. Using the criteria of uncorrected distance vision of 20/40 or better combined with near vision of J3 or better, 77% of eyes with the Array met the combined criteria compared to 46% of eyes receiving the monofocal IOL. As with other MIOLs, loss of contrast sensitivity at low testing levels was statistically significant. Eyes with normal-sized resting pupils (2.5 to 4.0) exhibited 0.6 to 0.9 line reduction in Snellen acuity at low contrast levels. Statistically significant differences in symptom rating scores between Array patients and monofocal controls were observed at 1 year for reports of difficulty with halos (15% versus 6%), glare/flare (11% versus 12%), and blurred vision (4% versus 1%). In spite of these differences, patient satisfaction scores for Array patients were high (95% reported that they were moderately to very satisfied with their surgery).[24]

The study protocol required surgeons to always aim for postoperative emmetropia in each eye. Therefore, postoperative monovision and/or intentional low postoperative astigmatism could not be employed to improve outcomes for monofocal eyes. This was necessary because the surgeon and clinical staff were unaware as to which lens was to be implanted, the Array or the monofocal IOL. Therefore, tailoring the surgery to a specific IOL type was not possible.

An interesting subset in this study looked at the effect the Array had on driving ability. The thought was that driving evaluations may help to determine just what adverse consequences loss of contrast sensitivity and halos might produce. Bilaterally implanted Array patients and monofocal control patients were evaluated while behind the wheel of an automobile driving simulation unit at the University of Iowa. The driving performance of the patients participating in this study was evaluated with a variety of road and weather conditions, such as nighttime driving with glare and fog. The results of this exercise showed that even though there were occasional situations in which monofocal patients did better (four of the 30 measures of performance), multifocal patients still performed within the safety guidelines. This suggests that the degree of reduction of low-contrast acuity and the greater incidence of halos at night with the Array MIOL may not necessarily translate into poor visual function.

The Array IOL represents the first real "proving ground" for MIOLs. As this multifocal lens continues to be successful, additional multifocal lens designs and enhancements of the Array lens are sure to follow.

Maximizing the Benefits of the Array

Since the Array FDA approval, a number of lessons have already been learned. Patient satisfaction with MIOLs is most likely to occur when:

1. Surgeons begin to consider cataract surgery to be a refractive procedure and that poor uncorrected near vision after cataract surgery is an undesirable result.
2. Office systems are in place to improve IOL calculation accuracy using precise biometry methods and the latest IOL calculation formulas.
3. Surgeons take advantage of the latest technology and techniques in cataract extraction.
4. Surgeons utilize surgical techniques to reduce unwanted astigmatism.
5. Surgeons and their staff monitor the results of IOL calculations and postoperative astigmatism, follow binocular uncorrected distance and near vision for all cataract surgery patients, and continually attempt to improve in all these areas.
6. Surgeons and clinical staff adjust the inclusion and exclusion criteria for patient selection as they become more familiar with this new technology.
7. Patients have reasonable expectations and understand that, as with any new visual system, the process of visual cortical adaptation is necessary before optimal results can be achieved.

References

1. Weale R. Presbyopia toward the end of the 20th century. *Surv Ophthalmol.* 1989; 34:15-30
2. Schachar R. Is Helmholtz's theory of accommodation correct? *Ann Ophthalmol.* 1999;31(1):10-17.
3. Wallace RB. *Multifocal Vision After Cataract Surgery.* Philadelphia, Pa: Rapid Science Publishers; 1998; 66-70.
4. Verzella F, Calossi A. Multifocal effect of against-the-rule myopic astigmatism in pseudophakic eyes. *Refract Corneal Surg.* 1993;9:58-61.
5. Sawusch M, Guyton D. Optimal astigmatism to enhance depth of focus after cataract surgery. *Ophthalmology.* 1991;96:1025-1029.
6. Cumming JS, Kammann J. Experience with an accommodating IOL. *J Cataract Refract Surg.* 1996;22:1001
7. Hara T, Hara T, Yasuda A, Yamada Y. Accommodative intraocular lens with spring action. Part 1. Design and placement in an excised animal eye. *Ophthalmic Surgery.* 1990;21:128-133.
8. Hara T, Hara T, Mizumoto Y, Yasuda A, Yamada Y. Accommodative intraocular lens with spring action. Part 2. Fixation in the living rabbit. *Ophthalmic Surgery.* 1992;23:632-635.
9. Boerner C, Thrasher B. Results of monovision correction in bilateral pseudophakes. *Am Intra-Ocular Implant Soc J.* 1984;10:49-50.
10. Keates R, Pearce J, Schneider R. Clinical results of the multifocal lens. *J Cataract Refract Surg.* 1987;13:557-560.
11. Ravalico G, Baccara F, Rinaldi G. Contrast sensitivity in multifocal intraocular lenses. *J Cataract Refract Surg.* 1993;19:22-25.
12. Wallace RB. 3M diffractive multifocal intraocular lens. In: Maxwell WA, Nordan LT, eds. *Current Concepts of Multifocal Intraocular Lenses.* Thorofare, NJ: SLACK Incorporated; 1991: 69-75.

13. Simpson MJ. The diffractive multifocal intraocular lens. *European J Implant Ref Surg.* 1989; 1:115-121.

14. Lindstrom R. Food and Drug Administration study update—One year results from 671 patients with the 3M multifocal intraocular lens. *Ophthalmology.* 1993;100:91-97.

15. Gimbel H, Sanders D, Raanan M. Visual and refractive results of multifocal intraocular lenses. *Ophthalmology.* 1991;98:881-888.

16. Auffarth G, Hunold W, Breitenbach S, Wesendahl T, Mehdorn E. Long-term results for glare and contrast sensitivity in patients with diffractive, multifocal intraocular lenses. *European J Implant Ref Surg.* 1994;6:40-45.

17. Bellucci R, Giardini P. Pseudoaccommodation with the 3M diffractive multifocal intraocular lens: a refraction study of 52 subjects. *J Cataract Refract Surg.* 1993;19:32-35.

18. Knorz M. Results of the True Vista bifocal IOL European multicentre study. *European J Implant Ref Surg.* 1992;4:245-248.

19. Knorz M, Aron-Rosa D, Claessens D, Seiberth V, Munch D. Vision with the True Vista bifocal IOL. *European J Implant Ref Surg.* 1992;4:95-98.

20. Shoji N, Shimizu K. Clinical evaluation of a 5.5 mm three-zone refractive multifocal intraocular lens. *J Cataract Refract Surg.* 1996;22:1097-1101.

21. Knorz M, Koch D, Marinez-Franco C, Lorger C. Effect of pupil size and astigmatism on contrast acuity with monofocal and bifocal intraocular lenses. *J Cataract Refract Surg.* 1994;20:26-33.

22. Steinert R, Post C, Brint S, et al. A prospective, randomized, double-masked comparison of a zonal-progressive multifocal intraocular lens and a monofocal intraocular lens. *Ophthalmology.* 1992;99:853-860.

23. Steinert R, Aker B, Trentacost D, Smith P, Tarantino N. A prospective comparative study of the AMO Array zonal-progressive multifocal silicone intraocular lens and a monofocal intraocular lens. *Ophthalmology.* 1999;106:1243-1255.

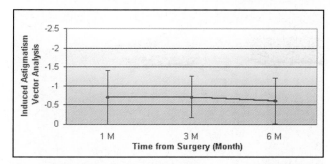

Figure 10-9c. Induced vector astigmatism shown over time after 3 mm sutureless IOL exchange.

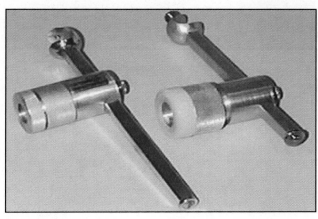

Figure 10-10. Practice device to hold eyes at the slit lamp for slit lamp astigmatic incisions (Eduardo Arenas, Trans. 21 no. 100-20 70, Piso, Bogata, DE Colombia).

al surgery. One good method of rehearsal is with a special device that holds an eyebank or pig eye in position to practice the technique. This device is available from Eduardo Arenas (Trans. 21 no. 100-20 70, Piso, Bogata, DE Colombia) and should be used prior to clinical implementation of the technique (Figure 10-10). The device clamps the eyebank or pig eye in and elevates its pressure. It then clamps on the side support of the slit lamp (Figure 10-11). With this device in place, the surgeon is able to practice both marking and incisions at the slit lamp. The difference between slit lamp surgery and surgery in the OR is mainly in the way the surgeon's hand and patient's eye are stabilized and the movement of the knife. In the OR, the hand is stabilized at the wrist and moves. At the slit lamp, the arm is stabilized by the elbow down on the table and the wrist at the headrest (Figures 10-12a and b). The hand is then kept relatively fixed and movements are accomplished primarily with the fingers. It is possible to lift the elbow off the table and move either the wrist and/or arm, but this results in less stability and untoward movements of the knife are accordingly more likely. In general, we suggest maintaining the stable positioning of the hand and elbow and using the patient's eye movements to move from one location to another. Specifically, the patient is asked to move his or her eye to make the appropriate incisions possible. To actually make the incisions, it is important to note that the movements are made with the fingers and that the fingers are not locked. To properly make the movements required for the incisions, the fingers should be formed like a "bellows," allowing easy movement of the knife (Figures 10-13a and b).

The easiest incisions to make are for against-the-rule astigmatism, since the incisions require a simple up-down sweep to create. Slightly more difficult are incisions for with-the-

Figure 10-11. Photo of the device clamped onto a slit lamp.

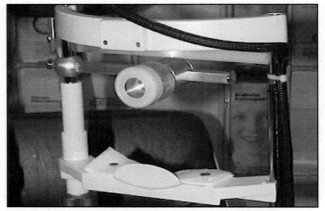

Figure 10-12a. Demonstration of proper stabilization of the arm with the elbow against the table and wrist against the chin rest for slit lamp astigmatic incisions.

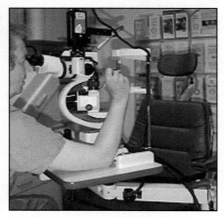

Figure 10-12b. Illustration of proper stabilization of the arm with the elbow against the table and wrist against the chin rest for slit lamp astigmatic incisions.

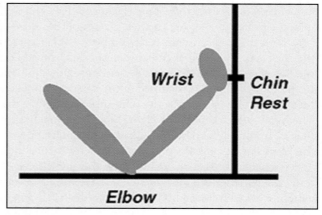

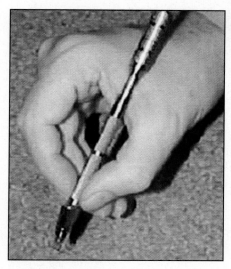

Figure 10-13a. Demonstration of proper grasp of a diamond knife to allow a "bellows" action of the fingers to move the knife for slit lamp astigmatic incisions.

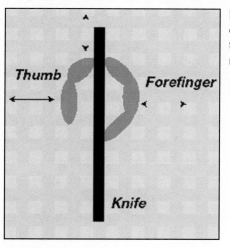

Figure 10-13b. Illustration of proper grasp of a diamond knife to allow a "bellows" action of the fingers to move the knife for slit lamp astigmatic incisions.

rule astigmatism, in which the lower incision is easily created and the patient is asked to look downward to complete the second incision. Care must be taken that the patient looks straight downward, since a slight deviation to the right or left will result in asymmetrical incisions. Oblique astigmatism can be the most challenging and requires particular care in attaining the proper axis (Figures 10-14a through c). We operate on the keratometric values and axis and will make every effort to align the manifest refraction with the keratometric values. Prior to the procedure, we refract the patient and leave the refraction in the phoropter in clear view near the patient's head. Alignment of the axis, particularly in oblique astigmatism, is therefore facilitated by observation of the axis in the phoropter and reference to the patient's eye (Figures 10-15a and b). The incisions are created by movement of the patient's eye to the proper position, with the "bellows" movement of the fingers for both incisions.

This technique is simply an adaptation of the technique used in the OR. We anesthetize the cornea with proparicaine used two to three times in a 5-minute period prior to the pro-

Figure 10-14a. Illustration of the easiest form of correction of astigmatism at the slit lamp for against-the-rule astigmatism.

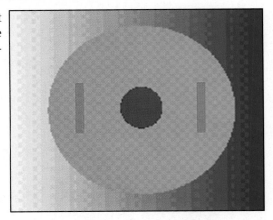

Figure 10-14b. Illustration of the slightly more difficult form of correction of astigmatism at the slit lamp for with-the-rule astigmatism.

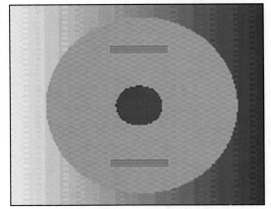

Figure 10-14c. Illustration of the most difficult form of correction of astigmatism at the slit lamp for oblique astigmatism.

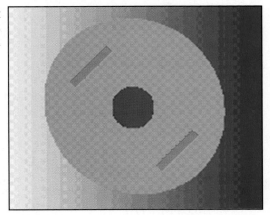

cedure. The decision to perform the incisions is usually made at the visit. The issue is discussed with the patient and a consent is obtained while in the room. The issue of postoperative adjustments is always discussed prior to the initial procedure, and the need for astigmatic enhancement usually comes as no surprise. Just as in topical anesthesia for cataract surgery, the mindset of the patient is important to the comfort and success of the procedure.

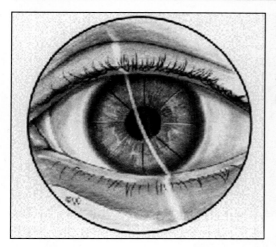

Figure 10-15a. Illustration of the technique to identify the proper axis of astigmatic correction by comparison of the slit lamp beam directed on the cornea to the phoropter situated beside the patient's head.

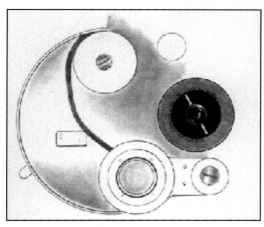

Figure 10-15b. Illustration of the technique to identify the proper axis of astigmatic correction by comparison of the slit lamp beam directed on the cornea to the phoropter situated beside the patient's head.

While enough time must be given for the anesthetic drops to take effect, excessive time cannot be taken to avoid unnecessary anxiety. Usually, the assistant is left in the room to give the drops, obtain the consent, and answer any minor questions. The patient is seated comfortably at the slit lamp and advised to keep the head against the headrest and chin down with mouth closed. The patient is asked to look directly ahead, either at a spot on the slit lamp or at the surgeon's contralateral ear. The assistant digitally retracts the lids, the patient is marked, and the incisions are made in relatively quick order. We use a 7 mm optical zone (OZ) and a gentian violet marking pen to mark the OZ centered on the pupil.

There are three important aspects to the incisions: depth, position (or optical zone), and length. We use an Osher diamond knife (Duckworth & Kent, London, England) with the head tilted at 45 degrees to allow good visualization of the knife blade at the slit lamp (Figures 10-16a through c). The diamond knife is set at 0.5 mm without regard to pachymetry, and arcurate incisions are created according to our published nomogram[6] to give an approximate corneal depth of 80%. We have found that deeper incisions lead to corneal instability and progressive corneal effect.[6] Again, to maximize corneal stability, we try to limit incision length to less than 60 degrees. A slight undercorrection is always advisable since retreat-

Figure 10-16a. Clinical slit lamp photograph of visualization obtained at the slit lamp with the angled diamond knife.

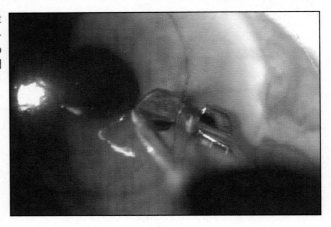

Figure 10-16b. Illustration of an angled diamond knife.

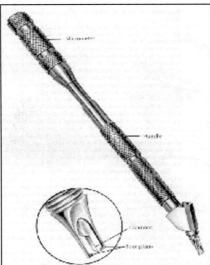

Figure 10-16c. Illustration of the obstruction of vision with a straight handled diamond knife versus the angled diamond knife.

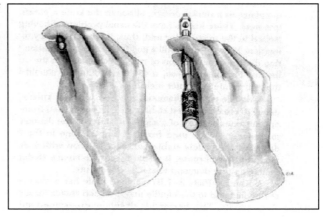

ment is just as simple as the original procedure. Afterward, we use Tobradex for 4 to 7 days, and the visual improvement is usually immediate. In usual cases, the patient will experience a two to three line visual improvement before leaving the office.

Summary

Enhancement after lens exchange or cataract surgery is not only possible but also simple and relatively easy to incorporate into the standard postoperative visits. The issue of spherical error after lens exchange occurs early in the postoperative course and once resolved, should not return as a significant problem over the medium to long run. In general, almost all hyperopic errors should be considered for revision since they impact reading vision, but fortunately they are much less common than myopic errors caused by excessive pressure in the measurement of axial length. It is important, as with all refractive surgeries, that periodic review of the results be performed to identify systematic problems in preoperative or operative management. Some good examples include policies concerning who actually performs the preoperative measurements and calculations. In our office, a single person is entrusted with this duty with a specified backup, both of whom I have personally trained. If neither of these are available, the patient is either asked to return on a different day or I perform the measurement. Difficult measurements, such as with excessive eye movement and/or dense lens opacities, are reviewed personally while the patient is present and before the case is calculated and accepted. If a new technician is being trained, I repeat all measurements for the first month until I am satisfied that the accuracy is acceptable. We have had situations in which other staff members were called to perform preoperative testing for lens surgery, and while in many cases the results were acceptable, in general the overall result was unacceptable. In addition, we perform keratometry measurements on the same machine, a Humphrey autokeratometer, and never rely on measurements from computed corneal topography. We have found that autokeratometry results from autorefractors can be operator dependent. If this instrument is selected, we would again recommend a single operator and preferably the same machine. Rounding mistakes can sometimes be a source of error, so we have an open-door policy concerning any question about individual cases and the proper decision before proceeding to surgery.

These policies might at first seem unnecessarily complex and demanding of the surgeon's time, but we believe refractive outcomes demand this level of effort. Every link in the chain of surgery can potentially cause a loss of quality and diminished refractive outcomes. Refractive surgery is a state of mind, not only for the surgeon but indeed for the entire staff, and they must be made a part of the continuing progress toward perfection. To those who say these procedures are too time-consuming for a busy practice, we respond that we perform well in excess of 1000 lens procedures per year and that these numbers do not prevent a smoothly functioning office. In fact, with our office automation software, Visual Office (Buzard Computer Solutions, Las Vegas, Nev), we are able to return outcome analyses virtually on demand, hold monthly office meetings on the refractive outcomes of our patients and discuss how we might be able to improve the results of outliers. This open interchange between staff and the office commitment that it implies are the key to the successful outcome of any refractive operation. The reward for this vigilance will be improved outcomes, happier patients and staff, and an increased volume of patients.

References

1. Buzard K, Shearing S, Relyea R. Incidence of astigmatism in a cataract practice. *J Cataract Refract Surg.* 1988;4(5):173-178

2. Merlin U. Curved keratotomy procedure for congenital astigmatism. *J Cataract Refract Surg.* 1987;3:92-97.

3. Shepherd JR. Induced astigmatism in small incision cataract surgery. *J Cataract Refract Surg.* 1989;15(1):85-8

4. Budak K, Friedman NJ, Koch DD. Limbal relaxing incisions with cataract surgery. *J Cataract Refract Surg.* 1998;24(4):503-8.

5. Talamo JH, Stark WJ, Gottsch JD, et al. Natural history of corneal astigmatism after cataract surgery. *J Cataract Refract Surg.* 1991;17(3):313-8.

6. Buzard KA, Laranjeira E. Clinical results of arcuate incisions to correct astigmatism. *J Cataract Refract Surg.* 1996; October:1062-1069.

7. Price RW, Grene RB, Marks RG, et al. Astigmatism reduction clinical trial: a multicenter evaluation of the predictability of arcuate keratotomy: evaluation of the surgical nomogram predictability. *Arch Ophthalmol.* 1995;113:277-282.

8. Duffey RJ, Jain VN, Tchah H, et al. Paired arcuate keratotomy; a surgical approach to mixed and myopic astigmatism. *Arch Ophthalmol.* 1988;106:1130-1135.

9. Thornton SP. Astigmatic keratotomy: a review of basic concepts with case reports. *J Cataract Refract Surg.* 1990;16:430-435.

10. Gills JP. The implantation of multiple intraocular lenses to optimize visual results in hyperopic cataract patients and under powered pseudophakes. Best Papers of Session, 1995. Symposium on Cataract IOL and Refractive Surgery Special Issue. *J Cataract Refract Surg.* 1996.

11. Gayton JL, Raanan MG. Reducing refractive error in high hyperopes with double implants. In: Gayton JL, ed. *Maximizing Results: Strategies in Refractive, Corneal, Cataract and Glaucoma Surgery.* Thorofare, NJ: SLACK Incorporated; 1996.

12. Gills JP. Multiple intraocular lens implantation. In: Gills JP, Fenzl R, Martin RG, eds. *Cataract Surgery: The State of the Art.* Thorofare, NJ: SLACK Incorporated; 1997.

13. Holladay JT, Gills JP, Leidlein J, Cherchio M. Achieving emmetropia in extremely short eyes with two piggyback posterior chamber intraocular lenses. *Ophthalmology.* 1996;103:1118-23.

14. Buzard KA. Deepening of incisions after radical keratotomy using the "tickle" technique. *J Refract Surg.* 1991;7:5:348-55.

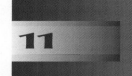

A-Scan Instrumentation and IOL Calculations

Brannon Aden, MD
Miles H. Friedlander, MD, FACS

Background and Introduction

As the science and technology of cataract extraction has evolved from couching centuries ago, to intracapsular extraction without intraocular lens (IOL) implantation, to modern small-incision phacoemulsification with IOL implantation, so too have evolved the expectations of both the ophthalmologist and the patient. In the past, the goal of surgery was for a good visual outcome; today, the goal is for a good refractive outcome. In the modern cataract surgeon's practice, patients expect to have a specific predicted final refraction, which in many instances is plano. Thanks to modern science, the technology for removing cataracts and improvements in IOL power calculation formulas that accurately preoperatively predict final postoperative refraction is a common reality. In some practices, clear lens extraction with aphakic IOL implantation, as well as the use of implantable or phakic IOLs, are being used as alternatives to keratorefractive surgery. As refractive phacoemulsification emerges as the standard, it is imperative for every cataract surgeon to have a solid working knowledge of the factors involved in the calculation of IOL power, common sources of measurement and calculation error, and an understanding of the performance of the various types of IOL designs and materials. This chapter has been designed to provide this information in simple and clinically applicable terms.

The average refractive power of the eye is approximately 60 diopters (D) of converging power with the anterior and posterior surfaces of the cornea accounting for an average of approximately 45 D and the lens accounting for the remaining 15 D. The earliest methods of cataract extraction surgery left the patient without a converging lens inside the eye. Harold Ridley, MD implanted the first IOL in London in 1949. His revolutionary opinion at the time, that "the cataract operation without a replacement lens was an incomplete, only half-finished operation,"[1] seems superfluous to the modern day cataract surgeon; however, it was not until the late 1960s to early 1970s that IOLs were routinely implanted. Even then, those that were used were of a standard power based on the above power averages. There was no attempt whatsoever made to control the final postoperative refraction. The first IOL that Ridley implanted was made of polymethylmethacrylate (PMMA), was implanted between the iris and anterior lens capsule, and was implanted 3 months following the original extracapsular cataract extraction procedure. The lens he used also resulted in a 14 D myopic over-correction. At that time, there was no such thing as an A-scan, which we rely upon so heavily today to calculate IOL power. With the advent of easy-to-use and relatively accurate ultrasonic biometry in the 1970s, direct measurement of the axial length of the eye became not only possible but was also surprisingly accurate. Shortly following the introduction of the A-scan came the "modern" era in IOL calculation technology. Many different ophthalmologists derived a variety of formulas, which they used to attempt to predict what power of implant lens would be needed inside the eye to eliminate the need for "cataract glasses."

If the axial length of the globe (distance from anterior corneal vertex to fovea), the index of refraction of aqueous/vitreous, the corneal power, and the location of the lens within the eye (this is essentially equivalent to anterior chamber depth) are known, then the refractive power of the lens needed to achieve emmetropia (or any other desired ametropic refraction) can be calculated. If the preoperative prediction of final postoperative refraction is to be accurate, then obviously the measurements taken to obtain each of the variables factored into any given IOL calculation formula, as well as the formula itself, must also be accurate. Any errors introduced into the equation, either as the result of an inherent formula weakness or of a measurement error, will be an additive in an algebraic fashion. Errors of the same sign will reinforce each other, and errors of opposite sign will cancel each other out. It is therefore essential for the cataract surgeon to eliminate as many sources of error as possible in order to best be able to control the patient's final refractive state and to avoid large refractive surprises.

As mentioned, there are a variety of potential sources for error in the calculation of IOL power, and they all fall into the general categories of either systematic error or random error. Systematic error occurs as the result of a weakness in the formula used or an inherent weakness in a measurement technique. For example, using an A-scan with a contact style probe results in slightly shortening the axial length measurement as the result of depressing the cornea, even in the hands of the most experienced technician. If, however, this error is consistent over time, the surgeon's results will always vary from the predicted value by the same margin and can thus be accounted for empirically by the surgeon. Systematic error is difficult to control, but due to the repetitive nature of such errors, tends to be less problematic in terms of overall accuracy of preoperative IOL power predictions. Rarely do large refractive surprises occur as the result of systematic error. On the other hand, random error is a much more problematic, as well as common, culprit in introducing significant error into the results of an IOL power calculation. The presence of a staphyloma, for example, whose exact location relative to the visual axis as measured by an A-scan, may be uncertain. Interpreting the A-scan of a patient with such a problem increases the probability of introducing random error into the calculation equation. Random error by definition does not occur often or with any degree of predictability. For the calculation of IOL power, errors (whether random or systematic) may result from measurement error, from unanticipated surgical effect, from weakness of the calculation formula, and rarely from equipment manufacturer error. Again, any one source of error will produce an additive effect when combined with any other type of error, making it critical to eliminate as many potential errors as possible when making a preoperative prediction of IOL power.

tion of IOL power, with this error being proportionately greater in significance for extreme-ly short eyes since any measurement error represents a larger proportion of the total per-centage of the axial length. A measurement error of only .25 mm results in a 1 D refractive error postoperatively. The presence of staphylomas in extremely myopic eyes is the most common reason for measurement error in long eyes, as it is often difficult to know where the fovea lies within the staphyloma. In short eyes, the anterior segment is very often of normal dimensions, while the posterior segment is proportionately much smaller than normal. Additionally, for short eyes, the overall tolerance for error is less than that for normal to abnormally long eyes because any deviation represents a greater proportion of the axial length.

Postoperative changes in axial length have also been suggested as a possible source of error with respect to axial length and the prediction of final refraction; however, various clinical studies have resulted in conflicting data as to whether this is of any clinical impor-tance.[8] The current standard of care is to apply the preoperative axial length measurement to the IOL calculation formula since a means of accurately predicting the postoperative axial length is not yet available.

Anterior Chamber Depth

In the formulation of the earliest theoretical IOL calculation formulas, anatomic ACD and final position of the IOL were essentially equivalent since the IOLs were placed in the anterior chamber and supported by the iris. In modern cataract surgery, the ACD has come to refer to the final position of the IOL, or the distance from the posterior vertex of the cornea to the anterior surface of the IOL which, generally speaking, is just posterior to the plane of the iris. ACD may be either measured directly using a pachymeter or calculated by a method described by Fyodorov.[3] Anatomic ACD is subject to variability due to the fol-lowing anatomic and physiologic factors: with age, the ACD grows shallower, at approxi-mately 0.1 mm per decade; with increasing myopia, ACD deepens by 0.06 mm per diopter.[8] The surgical ACD may be influenced by any of the following:
- The surgeon's operating style
- The type of lens used
- Wound closure technique
- Postoperative pharmacologic management[18]

An error of 0.1 mm in the preoperative estimation of ACD results in a refractive error of 0.1 D.[8] Current trends rely upon IOL calculation formulas that use a predicted value for the final position of the IOL within the eye, rather than a precisely measured ACD. Over the course of the evolution of the IOL calculation formulas, the importance of the ACD to the accuracy of each of the formulas has varied but is probably no longer a necessary factor in predicting final postoperative refraction.[8]

Corneal Curvature

As previously mentioned, any and all errors made during the course of calculating IOL power are additive. Preoperative measurement of corneal curvature in order to calculate corneal power is yet another essential component of the eye's optical system, which must be accurately determined.

Modern keratometry technology produces very reliable results; however, as for any measurement used in the course of calculating IOL power, it is important to ensure that the readings make sense relative to the patient's physical exam. The importance of evaluating all measurement results cannot be overstated, especially those results that are different from what the examiner expects or that deviate from the normal range for the population. An error of 0.1 mm in measuring the radius of corneal curvature results in a 1.0 D refractive error. Aside from measurement error, probably the most common source of error in measuring corneal curvature is the failure to remove contact lenses long enough prior to examination (2 to 3 weeks is recommended). With modern small incision and sutureless surgical technique, there is negligible change in preoperative corneal power.

Two special situations should be mentioned: 1.) measuring corneal curvature in a patient undergoing cataract extraction and 2.) IOL implantation in combination with penetrating keratoplasty. Many studies have been carried out in an attempt to determine how best to deal with this situation, and to date, there remains no overwhelming consensus. The enormous variation in surgical technique and suture patterns from one surgeon to the next makes this a very difficult parameter to evaluate. Equally as challenging, perhaps, is the determination of corneal power in postrefractive surgery patients. To date, there is no "standardized" means of dealing with this scenario. It is interesting to note with respect to corneal power that the further from the population average of 43.1 D of corneal power, the more error is introduced in the process of IOL power calculation, with this error being greatest in eyes with flat corneas.[20] Interestingly, McEwan, et al found that eyes with the combination of axial hyperopia and flat corneas had the largest standard deviation in calculation error.

Axial Length Measurement

Reliable A-scan technology became available in the mid 1970s. A-mode ultrasonic biometry has traditionally been the most widely used means of determining axial length and, until recently, also the most accurate. The ability to accurately measure axial length revolutionized cataract surgery. Current immersion A-scan ultrasound technology allows for reproducibility (precision) in measurement to within ±0.1 mm. An error of 0.1 mm in axial length measurement results in a postoperative refractive error of 0.25 D.[8] Contact A-scan ultrasound is less precisely reproducible, with an average error of ±0.2 mm.

A-scan measurements may vary depending on the brand of machine used. They may also vary depending on whether a stand-off (traditionally using an immersion technique) or contact method is employed. Contact A-scan probes may potentially introduce error into axial length measurement as the result of the probe (which must touch the cornea), indenting the cornea, and thus shortening the distance between the anterior corneal vertex and the fovea. While there may be no potential to falsely shorten the globe by using an immersion technique in which the probe is placed in a water bath that surrounds the cornea, this technique remains much more difficult and time consuming to perform, since patients must be in a recumbent position.

Dr. Kurt Buzard uses a technique of axial length measurement that he termed "touch and go," which combines the immersion and contact methods. In this technique, a table-mounted A-scan is essential. The technologist floods the patient's eye with artificial tears and instructs the patient not to wipe the eye. The contact probe is then advanced toward the eye until a retinal spike is produced on the oscilloscope. This step is repeated and the gain

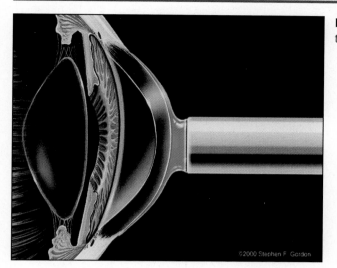

Figure 11-1. "Touch and go" technique.

©2000 Stephen F. Gordon

reduced to a sufficiently low level to still produce a series of full straight peaks. Because of the meniscus created by the copious amount of artificial tears, the probe is not in direct contact with the eye, but the ultrasonic waves still propagate through the ocular media. This technique combines the accuracy of the immersion technique (Figure 11-1) with the convenience and comfort of the contact technique while simultaneously eliminating the drawbacks of both techniques—namely, the mess and difficulty associated with placing a cup of water on a patient while in the recumbent position, and the underestimation of axial length caused by indenting the cornea. However, this technique requires a great deal of skill and experience on the part of the examiner.

Recently, a totally new technology for measuring axial length has been pioneered by Zeiss and Humphrey Instruments. The new IOL Master (Figure 11-2) uses the optical phenomenon of interference (partial coherence inferometry) to measure axial length. This technology is based on the principle that an interference signal will be produced if the measuring light is reflected by the retinal pigment epithelium (RPE). (A mode ultrasound measures sound waves reflected by the internal limiting membrane [ILM]). Because it employs light waves which, unlike sound waves propagate through air, this method of axial length measurement eliminates the need for both the contact as well as immersion techniques, which are necessitated by ultrasonography. The device is currently being tested at various centers around the country and will likely replace A-scan as the gold standard for axial length measurement. Not only does the device have the capacity to measure axial length, but it is also able to accurately measure both corneal power as well as anterior chamber depth, all in a single sitting. Preliminary results indicate that its accuracy is superior to that of all methods of A-scan. Best of all, it allows the patient to be seated for an exam that takes only 1 to 2 minutes to perform.

Regardless of the type of biometer used to determine axial length, human error remains the most important source of measurement error, making a skilled technician and a cooperative patient far more important in minimizing error and variability than the style of machine used. The immersion, contact, and touch and go methods all require the skill of a technician to maximize both accuracy and precision in measurement. Unfortunately, patient cooperativeness is very difficult to control or change. Most cataract patients are eld-

Figure 11-2. The Zeiss IOL Master.

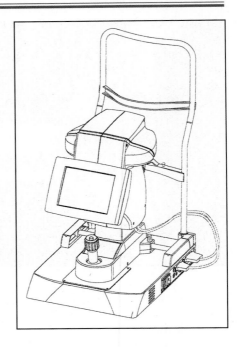

erly, and many have difficulty remaining still for the duration of the examination. The use of any instrument that stabilizes the patient's head, such as a table-based machine with a chin and forehead rest, helps to minimize error caused by movement of the patient. The advantage of the new IOL Master is two-fold: very little skill on the part of the examiner is required and the patient is able to sit comfortably in front of the machine for an exam that takes only a minute or two to perform.

Because the A-scan remains the gold standard at present for axial length measurement, it is important to mention the A-scan oscilloscope readout and what constitutes a reliable axial length measurement.

A good A-scan will have the following (essential) characteristics, shown in Figure 11-3:

1. A tall, straight corneal peak.
2. An anterior lens capsule peak reaching at least 90% of maximum height.
3. A posterior lens capsule peak reaching to between 50% and 75% of maximum.
4. A retinal spike whose rise is straight and forms a 90-degree angle with the baseline.
5. Few to no echoes in the vitreous cavity.
6. Orbital fat echoes posterior to the retinal spike.

If any of these characteristics are missing, the scan should be repeated until a good scan is obtained. The scan should then be repeated on the fellow eye and used as a control. Any discrepancy between the two eyes should then be explained before accepting the measurement as accurate.

A poor A-scan may exhibit any or all of the following, as illustrated in Figure 11-4.

1. Low anterior lens capsule peak with narrow anterior chamber depth.
2. Very low posterior lens capsule peak.
3. Aberrant echoes in the vitreous, or "chatter."
4. Poor rise of retinal echo.

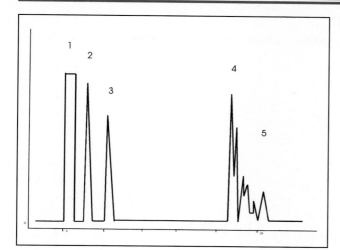

Figure 11-3. A good A-scan.

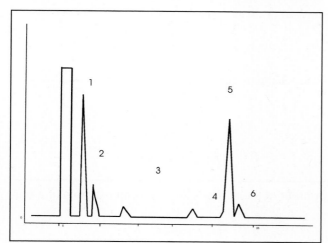

Figure 11-4. A poor A-scan.

5. Low retinal peak.
6. Absence of orbital fat echoes.

In the case of both Figures 11-3 and 11-4, the schematic A-scan oscilloscope printout depicts that which might be obtained using a contact method of measurement. The printout obtained using an immersion measurement technique differs from these only in that there will be two corneal spikes—the first representing the anterior surface and the second representing the posterior surface. Since a contact probe, by definition, is touching the anterior surface of the cornea, the two surfaces are represented together by a single spike.

In speaking with several A-scan technicians, all of whom are employed by high-volume cataract surgeons and all of whom have more than 15 years of experience measuring axial length, not surprisingly they report that they "just know" when they have obtained a reliable axial length measurement. They report a variety of observations that contribute to "just knowing," which includes:

*   Whether or not the patient was still and able to fixate on the target
*   The spikes on the oscilloscope

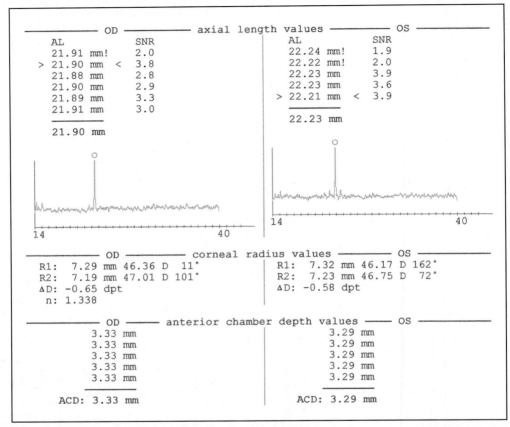

Figure 11-5. This oscilloscope printout of the author's left eye is an example of a reliable A-scan.

- The variability from one reading to the next
- The technician's evaluation of his or her own steadiness

Pictured in Figures 11-5 and 11-6 are oscilloscope printouts from an axial length measurement of the author's right and left eyes made with the hand-held, contact-style probe of an Alcon Ocu-Meter A-scan.

Figure 11-7 shows the printout produced by the IOL Master. The tall spike represents the reflection of light off the retinal pigment epithelium (RPE). Unlike an A-scan, the cornea, anterior and posterior lens capsules, and retina do not appear on the printout. A tall, narrow spike produced on a scan with a high signal-to-noise ratio (SNR) (SNR >2) is a reliable A-scan. The computer determines this internally. The secondary maxima are the two medium-sized spikes equidistant on either side of the RPE spike. These spikes are the result of the light source used by the machine, so they are always constant and independent of the characteristics of the tissue being measured.

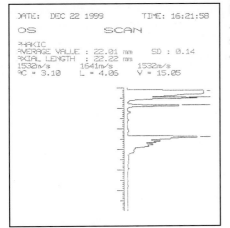

Figure 11-6. This oscilloscope printout of the author's right eye is an example of a poor A-scan. There is a large spike in the anterior vitreous.

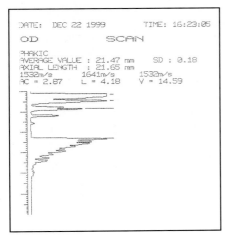

Figure 11-7. IOL Master printout of the author's measurements.

IOL Designs and Materials

While a lengthy discussion of the many different styles of IOLs and IOL materials is beyond the scope of this chapter, it is important to point out several principles that apply to the appropriate choice of IOL design. IOL design can account for IOL power errors of up to 1 or 2 D. The vast majority of lenses implanted today are either convex-plano, biconvex, or plano-convex. Plus and minus meniscus lenses (a few of which are still manufactured) have the greatest effect on final refraction (more than ±1 D respectively), whereas an equiconvex lens will have no effect. A convex-plano lens (whose curved surface is toward the cornea) will impart approximately 1 D of plus power to the IOL, whereas a plano-convex lens (curved surface toward the retina) will impart approximately 1 D of negative power to the IOL. Nonequiconvex biconvex lenses impart approximately ±0.50 D of additional power to an IOL, depending on whether the curved surface is toward the cornea or the retina.

The following practical scenario can be used to illustrate the point: A surgeon anticipates using an in-the-bag +20 D equiconvex lens but once in the operating room discovers that the power he needed for an emmetropic refraction was not available. He then discovers that the only other lenses available are plano-convex, then assuming that the A-constants are the same, the nonequiconvex lens would need to be +19.00 D in order to achieve emmetropia. Other factors, such as haptic angulation, also affect IOL power, and these effects may unpredictably vary depending on any one or more of the following factors:

- The size of the optic
- The vitreous pressure
- Haptic flexibility
- Contraction of the lens capsule

There are currently three basic types of IOL materials: PMMA, silicone, and acrylic. The choice of lens material is less a factor for power than for biocompatibility and performance; however, it is equally important to ensure a good visual/refractive outcome. For the normal nonallergic patient with a nondiseased eye, the choice of IOL materials can be left to the surgeon's preference. For eyes with silicone oil as a vitreous substitute, or for diseased eyes that may eventually require vitreoretinal surgery with silicone oil, heparin surface-modified 100% PMMA lenses should be used since this material has very low dispersive energy and tends to retard silicone oil adhesion to the lens.[21] Silicone oil tends to coat the surface of silicone lenses and to a lesser extent, acrylic lenses make subsequent posterior segment surgery very difficult or even impossible. Similarly, for uveitic eyes, heparin surface-modified 100% PMMA lenses should be used, not so much to lessen inflammation, but to prevent adhesion of protein to the lens.[22] Recently, many studies have been performed to determine what, if any, relationship exists between the lens material type and posterior capsule opacification (PCO). In a study by Ursell, et al in 1988, they found that acrylic lenses, and especially the Alcon AcrySof lens, were associated with significantly less PCO (median 11.75%) after 2 years than either silicone lenses (33.5%) or PMMA lenses (43.65%).[23] Interestingly, this remarkable difference has been attributed to the tacky surface of the AcrySof lens and its tendency to stick to the posterior capsule, preventing lens epithelial cells from proliferating behind the lens.

IOL Position

The location of any corrective lens relative to the the retinal photoreceptors is known to affect the refractive state of the eye. Figure 11-8 illustrates the various common locations for corrective lenses.

If a patient had a +10.00 D refraction in the spectacle plane (vertex distance of 15 mm), then a +11.76 D contact lens would be needed for emmetropia. The same principle applies with IOLs. The closer to the retina a plus lens is placed, the more powerful it must be to produce emmetropia. The converse is true for minus lenses—the closer they are placed to the retina, the less powerful they need to be to produce the same refraction. With respect to IOLs, there are essentially three places within the eye that they can be implanted: in the anterior iris plane, in the ciliary sulcus, and in the lens capsule. The more anteriorly the IOL (plus lens) is placed within the eye, the less powerful the lens will be in situ. For example, an IOL designed to go in the bag will produce a 1 D myopic overcorrection if that lens is placed 1 mm anterior to the lens capsule in the ciliary sulcus. For practical purposes, for every 1 mm that a lens is located away from its intended position, there will be a corresponding ±1 D refractive change.

12

Refractive Impact of the YAG Laser After Cataract Surgery

Daniéle Aron-Rosa, MD

Complications resulting from Nd:YAG Laser posterior capsulotomy include potential pitting of the intraocular lens (IOL), transient increase of intraocular pressure (IOP), opening of the hyaloid anterior face, cystoid macular oedema, uveitis, retinal hemorrhages, and retinal detachment.[1] However, most of them can be avoided even with a nanosecond laser by preventively treating the patient before and after Nd:YAG posterior capsulotomy. Apraclonidine 1% (Iopidine 1%) prevents IOP changes in 99% of the cases, and nonsteroidal anti-inflammatory drops prescribed from 1 day prior to capsulotomy to 1 week after are excellent prevention for inflammatory reactions and post-YAG cystoid macular edema (CME). Pitting of the lens and retinal hemorrhages are more dependent on the quality of the Nd:YAG laser—when the nanosecond YAG laser is multimode, the optical breakdown (OBD) does not occur constantly at low energy levels and generates possible risk of CME. When it does not occur, there can be retinal damages and increased risk of retinal detachment (5%). On the other hand, the threshold of OBD in the saline solution is much higher with multimode lasers, so generating extended shockwave effects can cause more drastic complications, such as CME, retinal detachment, pits on the lens, and secondary enlargements of the capsulotomy, which can be the cause not only of lens dislocation but also of changes in refraction.[2]

Opening the posterior capsule with picosecond (10 to 13 seconds) Nd:YAG or with femtosecond (10 to 15 seconds) Nd:YAG drastically reduces the rate of complications.[3] When the optical breakdown that is constantly obtained even in air at very low emergent energy levels (ie, in the microjoules range), the shock wave expansion is limited to 50 to 100 microns and the elevation of temperature is considerably reduced in time and surface extension. Pitting the lens and opening the anterior face of the hyaloid can be easily avoided, and the risk of retinal hemorrhages, CME, and retinal detachment is reduced to less than 0.01% (>1.75%). Morphologic changes may cause longitudinal displacement of in-the-bag implanted IOLs after posterior capsulotomy. However, no matter what laser is used, refraction and anterior chamber length modifications are more dependent on the material and design of the lens, the width of the anterior capsulorrhexis, and the size of the posterior capsule opening.

In a prospective study by Thornval and Naeser,[4] the refraction and the anterior chamber depth before and after nanosecond multimode Sharplan (Tel Aviv, Israel) YAG laser capsulotomy on 52 pseudophakic patients was studied. All the patients were implanted after planed extracapsular extraction, curvilinear continuous anterior capsulorrhexis, and in-the-bag implantation. All the lenses implanted were one-piece polymethylmethacrylate (PMMA) PCL biconvex or planoconvex with 7 to 6.5 mm optic diameter and overall length of 14 mm; the haptics of the lens were angled 10 degrees anteriorly. They were compared to a 44-patient pseudophakic group who had similar ECCE but no YAG laser capsulotomy.

The distance between the anterior corneal surface and the surface of the lens was measured optically with a modified Haag Streit type II pachymeter (Bern, Switzerland) attached to the slit lamp. After capsulotomy, the capsular opening was measured immediately and 5 weeks after using the Haag Streit slit lamp. The change in ACD was about 0.01 mm and no spectacle adjustment was necessary. They concluded that there was no significant change in the mean ACD or spherical equivalent refraction between two measurements of the capsulotomy group and control group, nor was there a statistically significant change in the mean values between the groups.

Mean capsulotomy diameter increased from 3.44 + 061 mm (+ SD) (range 2.15 to 4.68) immediately after YAG capsulotomy to 3.67 + 061 (range 2.00 to 5.20 mm) 5 weeks later. Thornval and Naesser concluded that the increase of 023 + 026 mm was statistically significant (P<1 x 10.7). More recently in 1999, Findl, et al[5] quantified position and the potential refractive modifications induced by Nd:YAG laser capsulotomy in three IOL styles with the Zeiss nanosecond YAG laser.

In their prospective study, the anterior chamber depth was measured by dual beam partial coherence interferometry (PCI) in 32 pseudophakic eyes with posterior capsular opacification before and immediately after Nd:YAG capsulotomy under mydriasis. The capsulotomy induced a backward IOL movement in all eyes, mean 25 microns (range 9 to 55 microns). It was more pronounced in eyes with plate haptic IOLs than with those of other styles. Precision of ACD by dual beam PCI was 4 microns. Changes in ACD correlated significantly with the capsulotomy size but not with the pre-YAG lens capsule distance. The larger the capsulotomy, the more backward the displacement of the lens. Also capsulotomy caused a backward movement of the IOL that was more pronounced with the plate haptic silicone IOLs than with the one-piece PMMA and the three-piece foldable IOL.

Since the magnitude of IOL movement in this study population was small, the hyperopic shift in refraction after capsulotomy was small and not clinically relevant. In a prospective study, we compared the effect of picosecond YAG laser capsulotomy on the changes in IOL position on two types of foldable IOLS: the plate haptic silicone STAAR AA 42 03V F in 30 eyes and the easy Kelios (Chauvin, France) three-piece foldable lens (optical diameter 6 mm, overall length 11.2 mm) in 30 eyes in a control group (60 patients) who had similar surgery and implants but no YAG.

All the patients had cataracts removed by phacoemulsification after continuous curvilinear capsulorrhexis. In all patients, anterior chamber depth was measured by dual beam partial coherence interferometry at 6 months after implantation, immediately after YAG capsulotomy, and 5 weeks after YAG. The measurements were done at similar dates for the non-YAG control group.

Our results partially corroborate those of Findl, et al.[5] The capsulotomy induced a backward movement of the IOL in all cases (Figure 12-1) at day 1. It varied from 10 to 28 microns for the three-piece foldable, and from 15 to 55 microns for the plate IOL. At 5 weeks after YAG, there was no significant change in the three-piece IOL position; however, there was a tendency for backward movement of the plate IOL (16 to 60 microns). The hyperopic shift in refraction immediately after capsulotomy was irrelevant and remained so

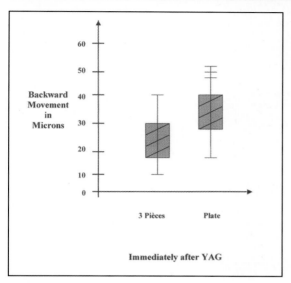

Figure 12-1. Anterior chamber depth varies from 10 to 28 microns for the 3-piece IOL and from 15 to 55 microns for the plate IOL.

5 weeks later; however, there was a mean hyperopic shift for the plate lenses, mean sphere equivalent 0.15 D (extreme 0.08 to 0.05), and two patients with a small anterior capsulorrhexis (inferior to 5 mm) and a mean induced astigmatism of 0.30 D. At 5 weeks, we did not notice any change in the capsulotomy size.

The Nd:YAG laser capsulotomy causes a backward movement of the IOL regardless of the type of implanted lens when precisely measured with the dual-beam partial coherence interferometer. The nature of the YAG laser influences the evolution of the capsulotomy size. If the laser is multimode, more energy is required and the importance of the shockwave causes secondary enlargement of the posterior capsulotomy. When the Nd:YAG is monomode, whether nano-or picosecond, it does not generate a substantial difference in the evolution of the size of the capsulotomy.

The foldable plate IOL demonstrates a tendency for backward displacement, mainly when the continuous circular capsulorrhexis (CCC) is narrow. Plate haptic IOLs tend to be compressed in the shrinking capsule and vault backward, resulting in increased capsular tension. When the capsule is released, there is less resistance and the lens vaults backward even more; if the capsular opening is large enough, they may dislocate in the vitreous.

Conclusion

Nd:YAG capsulotomy causes backward displacement of the IOL, which is significantly higher with plate haptic IOLs and in cases of large capsulotomies; however, it generates minimal refractive changes. It seems to be reasonable to recommend small, well-centered capsulotomies, mainly when the Nd:YAG is nanosecond and multimode with optical breakdown occurring at either high energy levels that will generate evolution and enlargement in the size of the posterior capsulotomy.

Figure 12-2. There is no significant difference in the backward movement of the IOL as compared to day 1.

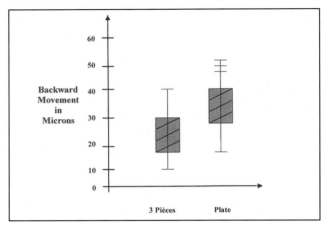

References

1.   Aron Rosa, D. *Pulsed YAG Laser Surgery.* Thorofare, NJ: SLACK Incorporated: 1983: 153.
2.   Aron Rosa D, Aron JJ, Griesemann M. Use of Nd:YAG laser to open the posterior capsule after lens implant surgery. *J Am Int Implant Soc.* 1980;6:352-354.
3.   Griesemann JC, Decroisette M. Thermal wave propagation and shock wave formation in optical breakdown. *J App Phys.* 1979;50:3915-3920.
4.   Thornaval P, Naeser K. Refraction and anterior chamber depth before and after Nd:YAG laser treatment for posterior capsule opacification in pseudophakic eyes. *J Cataract Refract Surg.* 1995;21:457-460.
5.   Findl O, Drexler W, Menapace R, et al. Changes in intraocular lens position after Nd:YAG capsulotomy. *J Cataract Refract Surg.* 1999;25:659-662.

Lens-Based Surgery After Corneal Refractive Surgery

Jean-Luc Febbraro, MD
Kurt A. Buzard, MD, FACS

Introduction

Since the widespread introduction of radial keratotomy (RK) and excimer laser keratectomy over the last two decades, corneal refractive surgery has been performed on several million patients throughout the world. As with everyone, these patients age and, at the very least, develop refractive changes related to the lens, often developing lens changes that impair best-corrected vision. These patients represent a special sort of health consumer and are very aware of changes in their vision. As a result, they often present with early cataracts, making evaluation even more challenging. Most patients were at least initially successfully treated with refractive surgery and sometimes no longer needed corrective lenses to reach emmetropia, although almost all of them have problems with reading and others have visual symptoms related to the original refractive surgery. Nearly all of these patients, two or three decades later, will develop cataracts and may be candidates for cataract surgery. As a result of the cataract formation and inevitable changes in the original corneal refractive procedure, particularly if it is radial keratotomy (RK), these patients often present with visual changes that must be sorted out with respect to cornea versus lens versus other problems, such as dry eye, diabetic retinopathy, macular degeneration, etc. In addition, their refraction may shift during the day, making evaluation on a single visit difficult. In fact, both uncorrected and best-corrected vision may change throughout the day. These patients are often highly motivated to see without correction and have the same expectations after the cataract procedure.

It would seem natural to consider these patients for cataract or clear lens procedures as a remedy to cataract and/or refractive problems and, in fact, we often do recommend this approach. This chapter will focus on the challenges that exist with respect to lens-based surgery in these patients. While these issues are often intimidating, in many cases, cataract or lens exchange surgery represents the best option for the patient. If the reader is surprised by the careful wording and circumspect recommendation for lens-based surgery, then the correct impression has been given. This chapter will focus on corneal refractive patients presenting for lens surgery and the many challenges these patients introduce. We will begin with the calculation of proper lens power, but we qualify at the outset that all methods are less than perfect and whatever lens one chooses, the patient and surgeon must often be prepared for a long relationship.

The accuracy of the postoperative refraction is an obvious area of problems after corneal refractive procedures because the optical properties of the eye have been permanently altered. In fact, refractive procedures such as RK, photorefractive keratectomy (PRK), or laser in situ keratomileusis (LASIK) flatten the central part of the cornea to correct myopia and, thus, change the asphericity of the cornea from a prolate shape to an oblate shape. This corneal modification is a source of inaccuracy for the measurement of the central keratometry and has an impact on intraocular lens power (IOLP) prediction.

Markovits reported a clinical case of a patient who had undergone radial keratotomy prior to cataract removal. The postoperative spherical equivalent was +0.25 diopter 9 months postoperatively, whereas the implanted intraocular lens (IOL) was 3 diopters (D) stronger than the IOL power calculated by using the mean standard keratometric value.[1] Koch and coauthors have found that standard keratometric readings tend to overestimate true corneal power and result in underestimation of the required IOL power.[2] Siganos and associates published a case of a patient who underwent PRK and subsequently required a cataract extraction in which the IOL power was undercorrected by 3.50 D.[3] Several methods can be used to measure corneal power in eyes that have undergone corneal refractive surgery. In addition to standard keratometry, other options, such as the refraction-derived keratometric value, the contact lens overrefraction method of Soper and Goffman, and computerized videokeratography, are also available.[4,5,6,7]

Along with the known problems of IOL power calculation, we feel there is much more to discuss with respect to these patients. They often present challenges to the surgeon with respect to patient expectations, refractive and pathologic diagnosis, postoperative care, and financial considerations if the diagnosis is indeed cataract formation. As we previously mentioned, the patient will inevitably compare the cataract surgery with the previous refractive surgery, both in terms of length of recovery and corrected and uncorrected visual acuity. Patients are often working or at the very least very active, and a prolonged recovery (which is almost inevitable in some cases) may both inconvenience the patient and lead to dissatisfaction with the surgery.

Virtually all previous RK patients have some amount of regular and irregular astigmatism, are often overcorrected, have some degree of diurnal variation and loss of contrast and glare, even without the formation of a cataract. When an early cataract is added, the additive loss of contrast can be significant, yet removal of the cataract removes only a portion of the problem. Since recovery is not complete, the patient may again be disappointed with the result. However, use of other corneal refractive procedures, such as LASIK may actually add to the loss of contrast while improving the refractive situation, possibly making the subjective vision worse. Additionally, the patient may not even realize that diurnal variation is one of the problems and, of course, the surgery will not improve and could potentially worsen the situation. Normally, a diurnal shift in vision begins with hyperopia in the morning, clearing around noon, and turning to myopia at night. While the shifts can be almost unnoticeable, they can also be as large as 2 D. Many patients have adapted to whatever changes occur, and if the patient is slightly over- or undercorrected, it will result in an upset of these changes—perhaps making it impossible to drive in the morning or read in the evening, which again may result in patient dissatisfaction.

Finally, after the surgery, the cornea will flatten for an undetermined amount of time, resulting in hyperopia that goes away slowly and may require the use of contact lenses or glasses for an undetermined amount of time. It may seem that we have introduced so many issues that it is virtually impossible to obtain a result that satisfies the patient, but in fact we perform both cataract and clear lens exchange surgery on previous RK patients regularly and with good success. The key to success is proper patient education and realistic goals for post-operative vision. Testing can give some insight but wide variability in terms of vision, and speed of recovery will exist from patient to patient—both surgeon and patient must accept this fact prior to any intervention.

In this chapter we will describe and analyze the different methods to evaluate the corneal power required in the IOL in eyes that have undergone corneal refractive surgery. We will also share our personal experiences and relate published studies in order to provide practical suggestions for increasing accuracy of IOL power calculation and improving patient satisfaction with lens-based surgery.

Preoperative Evaluation and Counseling

When a patient with a previous corneal refractive surgery presents, we will routinely obtain refraction, topography, and photokeratometry if he or she is new or has not been seen for some time. Of course, RK and to a lesser extent, astigmatic keratotomy, are the previous surgeries that are the most common in this circumstance and have the most issues with respect to corneal stability. As we mentioned, these patients are often accustomed to good uncorrected vision and often seek treatment for cataract at an early stage of development or for hyperopic shift with resulting blurred uncorrected vision. Examination of topography as well as photokeratometry can give some insight into the stability of the RK incisions and to the presence of irregular astigmatism that may complicate diagnosis. An example is seen in Figures 13-1, 13-2, and 13-3 in which both photokeratometry and computed topography show irregular astigmatism with breaking of mires and power shifts across the visual axis, which are the hallmark features of irregular astigmatism.[8] Patients with extremely small optical zones, epithelial inclusions in the incisions, more than eight radial incisions, and/or relaxing incisions that cross the visual axis are more likely to have irregular astigmatism and visual complaints are likely to be related to this problem rather than the lens (Figures 13-4, 13-5, and 13-6).

In patients with previous RK, we routinely note the time of examination and carefully question the patient concerning diurnal variability of vision. The pertinent questions are how long uncorrected distance vision is blurred in the morning, when best vision occurs during the day, and if distance vision again blurs at night. In a typically well-healed RK patient, mild blurring occurs for an hour in the morning and peaks about noon or 1 pm. The patient has a little trouble driving in the evening with slight blurring in good light but notices an improvement in reading vision in the afternoon. These symptoms may vary dramatically from patient to patient, and if the patient is complaining about vision or if surgery is contemplated, detailed understanding of these changes are essential to properly counsel him or her and to avoid a surgical solution for a problem that might not be surgical in nature. We will often ask the patient to return later in the day to document refraction, uncorrected vision, and reading vision at different times.

After examination and discussion with the patient, the surgeon should be able to answer the question, "What is the real complaint with vision?" Is it a reading problem during the entire day, only in the morning, or at different distances, such as for computer work? For morning reading problems, 1% pilocarpine given in the morning or night before can signif-

Figure 13-1. Breaking of mires on an eight-cut RK showing corneal instability and mild to moderate irregular astigmatism.

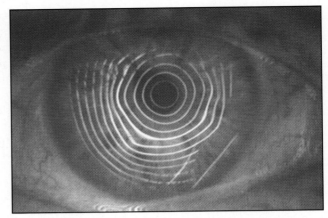

Figure 13-2. Breaking of mires with significant changes in power across the visual axis after 32-incision RK showing severe regular and irregular astigmatism resulting in 20/100 best-corrected vision.

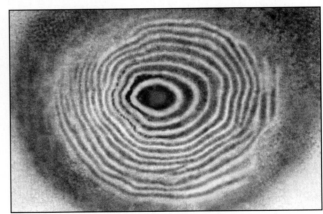

Figure 13-3. Inferior corneal perforation showing corneal instability and irregular astigmatism with a v-shaped microdihesence.

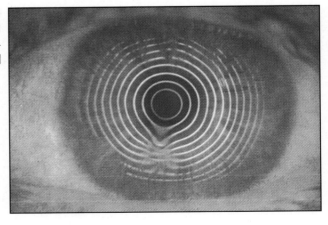

icantly improve morning blurring and blunt diurnal shifts in vision.[9] For more routine reading problems, simple magnifiers or monovision might be suggested. In the patient under age 50, we will perform hyperopic LASIK for monovision but routinely perform clear lens exchange in older patients with good success, since the endpoint is less critical and an initial hyperopic shift does not greatly inconvenience the patient in the short-term postopera-

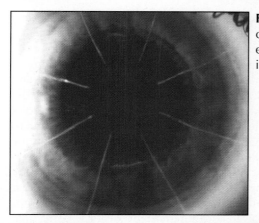

Figure 13-4. Stable appearance of an eight-cut RK with nonintersecting T-cuts without epithelial inclusions and no evidence of instability.

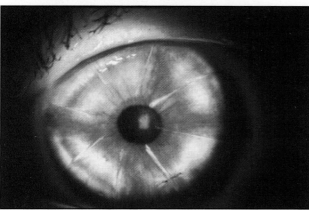

Figure 13-5. Eight-cut RK with epithelial inclusions and widened incisions, which are evidence of mild to moderate corneal instability.

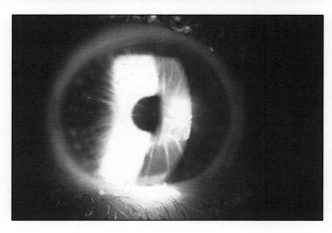

Figure 13-6. Thirty-two-incision RK showing evidence of severe corneal instability with a sub 3 mm optical zone, subepithelial fibrosis, and epithelial inclusion.

tive time period. We routinely test the monovision correction with a contact lens prior to surgery and find that these patients are more pleased with a larger monovision correction of 2 to 2.5 D. Remember that these patients were initially nearsighted and thus at a slightly higher risk for retinal detachment. We routinely ask all myopic patients undergoing clear lens exchange to obtain a visual field and retinal examination. We have found the Array multifocal IOL to be a poor choice in this circumstance due to the additive loss of contrast sensitivity.

If the patient complains of distance vision problems, are they just at certain times of the day or continuous? Is the problem merely diminished uncorrected vision or is best-corrected vision also affected? Again, morning blurring can be helped with 1% pilocarpine and evening glare can sometimes be treated with 0.1% to 0.25% pilocarpine, which we have the patient create with dilution of the pilocarpine and artificial tears. If the patient is overcorrected, try a contact lens to show him or her the potential vision throughout the day and to test whether other complaints arise. Even if the overcorrection is more than 1 to 2 D in the morning, avoid operating with less than 1 D at the time of best vision (usually early afternoon) and particularly if the vision is 20/40 at this point. Even though the patient may be very overcorrected at one point of the day, a refractive surgery will only shift the time that the patient is functional or turn a hyperope into a myope. Be realistic, even if the patient is not perfectly happy. Can the problem be resolved with intermittent spectacle correction, particularly for night driving? The patient with a drop in vision from 20/20 to 20/50 may demand a surgical solution and in some circumstances, it is appropriate to proceed, but the potential of extended recovery and an even bigger "short-term" decrease in uncorrected vision may make the experience unpleasant for surgeon and patient.

Calculation Methods of Corneal Power

Six different methods are available to estimate the corneal power of the eye that has undergone corneal refractive surgery and to adjust the power of the calculated IOL:

1. Keratometry
2. Refractive history
3. Contact lens
4. Computerized videokeratography
5. Assumption of a fixed addition to the IOL power
6. Intraoperative adjustment of IOL power

Keratometry

Standard keratometers measure a 3 mm diameter annulus to estimate the corneal power. They project a mire onto the corneal surface and measure the reflections of four corneal points 1.5 mm from the corneal apex. The diameter of the annulus depends on the radius of curvature of the cornea and increases as corneal curvature decreases. In unoperated eyes, keratometric readings have proven to be a reliable estimation of central corneal power. IOL calculations are based on keratometric readings and provide satisfactory refractive predictability and accuracy.

After RK, the central cornea flattens more than the paracentral cornea, and the midperipheral may steepen. The rate of change of the corneal curvature is increased at the inflection zone (paracentral knee).[10] Celikkol and coauthors have found that the inflection zone is located between 2.40 and 3.00 mm from the center of the ring.[11] If the inflection zone is within 3 mm, a standard keratometer measures a region of the cornea that is steeper than the flatter central cornea. The same authors have found that the keratometric reading was, on average, 1.76 D steeper than the ideal keratometric reading, and IOLs were consequently undercorrected by 2.32 D.

After PRK, flattening of the cornea is more homogeneous than after RK. However, the central cornea is also flatter than the peripheral cornea. As a consequence, the keratometric reading after PRK generates the same misleading information as after RK. The keratometric readings correspond to a more peripheral corneal zone and therefore give an erroneously steep reading of the effective central corneal curvature. After PRK, automated keratometry has been reported to underestimate the corneal power change by 20% to 25%.[12]

The inaccuracy of standard keratometry after RK or PRK results in an underestimation of the required IOL power. Published results have shown that refraction after cataract surgery following RK and PRK ranged from 1 to 6 D of hyperopia, despite aiming for emmetropia.[2,13] After RK, the hyperopic shift is particularly marked during the 3 to 6 months after cataract surgery. A transient corneal flattening causes this shift, which is more noticeable during the first week. This corneal flattening partially regresses over the following 3 to 6 months but still persists over time to a lesser degree. Corneal power overestimation and IOL power underestimation has been significantly correlated with the spherical equivalent change after PRK and the intended ablation depth during PRK.[13]

After RK, the acute hyperopic shift is probably linked to the corneal edema that is present after cataract surgery. MacRae and associates have found a correlation among the corneal swelling, corneal flattening, and diurnal fluctuations that occur in patients that have undergone RK.[14] Koch has found that corneal flattening had followed the same temporal pattern in a group of patients operated on for cataract after RK. In addition, the same author found that the severity of the early postoperative flattening decreased as the interval between RK and cataract surgery increased. The long-term healing of RK could blunt the edema and induce an acute hyperopic shift after cataract surgery.[2] The small amount of persistent hyperopic shift could be explained either by the persistence of the acute postoperative flattening or by the hyperopic shift that occurs in eyes that have undergone RK. In fact, the RK group showed that 43% of eyes changed in the hyperopic direction by 1 D or more between 6 months and 10 years after RK.[15]

It appears that the hyperopic shift after cataract surgery following RK is linked to mechanical instability of the cornea. In contrast, the hyperopic shift after PRK may be predominantly related to the change of the anterior surface curvature and to the reduction of corneal thickness.

Standard keratometers estimate the corneal power by measuring the anterior radius of curvature. The following formula is used to calculate the corneal power:

P = (n − 1) / r
P = corneal power (D)
n = refractive index
r = radius of curvature (m)

Keratometers use a refractive index of 1.3313. This refractive index is valid if the measured cornea is similar to Gullstrand's model. In this model, the refractive index characterizes a single refractive surface that represents both the anterior and the posterior surfaces of the cornea. After PRK, the cornea is not only flatter but also thinner. As a consequence, the radius of the anterior surface of the cornea is increased, but the distance between anterior and posterior surfaces of the cornea is decreased. Thus, the method of calculating corneal power from radius of curvature becomes inaccurate.[16,17]

More recently, LASIK has been performed on a large scale, and no published data is available today to show the IOLP implications after cataract surgery. However, this technique is theoretically similar to PRK in terms of corneal modification; in addition, it allows for the correction of higher degrees of myopia. For this reason, LASIK may further reduce the thickness of the cornea and may induce a larger miscorrelation between the anterior and posterior curvature of the cornea. Here again, the model eye would be insufficient to calculate corneal power from radius of curvature.[13]

Refractive History

The refractive history method has been devised by Holladay and requires the average keratometry prior to corneal refractive surgery. The refractive change is obtained by subtracting the postoperative from the preoperative spherical equivalent refraction.[18] This calculation needs to correct the vertex distance to the plane of the cornea. The following formula can be used:

Rc = Rs/(1-vRs)

where Rc = power (D) at corneal plane; Rs = power (D) at vertex (v) distance; V = vertex distance(in meters)

or

Rc = Rs/(1-0.0012Rs), assuming a spectacle distance of 12 mm.

For example, in an eye after RK:
- Preoperative average K reading 44 D
- Preoperative refraction -4.00 @ vertex 12 mm = -3.80 @ corneal plane
- Postoperative refraction -0.50 @ vertex 12 mm = -0.50 @ corneal plane

The change in refraction is calculated by algebraically subtracting the postoperative power from the preoperative power:

-3.80 – (-0.50) = -3.30 D

The estimated corneal power after RK is calculated by algebraically adding the change in refraction at the corneal plane to the preoperative corneal power:

44 + (-3.30) = 40.70 D
40.70 D is then used for the IOLP calculation

Refraction measurements improve if a long period of time has elapsed between refractive surgery and the keratometric reading. In addition, the postoperative refraction can be biased by the presence of a cataract.[19] Despite these limitations, the IOL power calculation method based on refractive history seems to be more reliable than the standard keratometric readings. Seitz and associates have shown that in comparison to this method, direct power measurements underestimate corneal flattening by 24% on average.[13] Celikkol and coauthors have found that the refraction-derived keratometric values induce only +0.15 + 0.52 D deviation from the ideal keratometric value, and the IOL powers calculated with these values are –0.16 + 0.49 D different than the ideal.[11]

However, the refractive history method requires the preoperative refraction and keratometry, and this data is often difficult to obtain as corneal refractive surgery is usually performed several decades before the cataract procedure. This method would be used more often if refractive surgeons systematically gave their patients a chart with preoperative keratometric readings, preoperative refraction, and a stable postoperative refraction at least 6 months after the refractive procedure.

Contact Lens Method

The effective corneal power after refractive surgery can be estimated by using the contact lens overrefraction method described by Soper and Goffman.[6] This method requires a manifest refraction (eg, -0.50 D SE) without a contact lens and then a repeat of the manifest refraction after placing a hard contact lens of known posterior curvature and power on the eye. If the refraction does not change (eg, -0.50 D SE) and the contact lens has no power and a 42 D base curve, the central corneal curvature is equal to the base curve of the contact lens. The estimated keratometric reading for IOL power calculation is 42 D. If the overrefraction is -1 D and the contact lens has a -0.25 D power and a 42 D posterior curve, the following calculation is used. The lens posterior curve is added to the lens power to obtain the total surface power of the diagnostic lens:

42 + (-0.25) = 41.50 D

The spherical equivalent of the overrefraction is added to the total power of the diagnostic lens:

41.50 + (-1.00) = 40.50 D

From this, the original refractive error is subtracted to obtain the effective corneal power:

40.50 − (-0.50) = 41.00 D

The effective corneal power used for IOL power calculation is 41 D.

The contact lens trial method allows for the estimation of the corneal power based on the manifest refraction of the patient. It has the advantage of not being dependent on the preoperative keratometry. However, this method may be problematic, as not all ophthalmologists have hard contact lenses available. Last but not least, this method may be severely inaccurate if the patient has a dense cataract and/or if the cataract induces a myopic shift.

Videokeratography

Computerized videokeratography is systematically used in refractive surgery today, not only during the preoperative screening but also for the surgical planning and the postoperative assessment of the refractive outcome and the ablation centration.[20,21]

Computerized keratography provides a detailed picture of the shape of the cornea by measuring thousands of points of the corneal surface. These measurements of corneal curvature are based on the projection of Placido discs with analysis of a Purkinje image. Videokeratography can measure the central corneal curvature overlying the entrance pupil.

Cuaycong and coauthors found that in patients that had undergone cataract extraction, computerized topography-derived keratometric values were more accurate than standard keratometric values.[22] They found that with the EyeSys corneal analysis system, the 3-mm zone average and the mean central corneal power were the most accurate. The mean central corneal power is defined as the average of all the values over 360 meridians of the central nine ring edges.

Celikkol and associates have found that with the TMS-1 (Tomey Technology, Cambridge, Mass), which is able to measure a smaller central zone than the EyeSys, the mean power in ring three gives the most accurate keratometric reading.[11] These studies revealed that computerized videokeratography could be advantageously used to calculate IOL power in patients that had undergone RK. Compared to standard keratometry, computerized keratography measures more points over a larger region of the central cornea and thus determines true corneal refractive power more accurately. In addition, significant differences may be relevant in keratomized patients. In these corneas, the postoperative shape has changed from prolate to oblate. Thus, videokeratography-derived keratometric readings may more accurately evaluate the effective corneal power than a standard keratometric reading that measures four points at an approximately 3-mm zone.

More recently, computerized videokeratography has been used to estimate the IOL power for cataract surgery after myopic PRK. Seitz and coauthors have not found more accurate information with corneal topography compared to standard keratometers. On average, the flattening of the cornea was underestimated by 20%. Topographic corneal powers have been significantly greater than the respective keratometric reading, have induced smaller IOLP values and, consequently, postoperative hyperopia after cataract surgery.[13] Quah and associates have published similar results noting that refraction after cataract surgery following PRK ranged from 1 to 6 D of hyperopia.[12] According to Odenthal and coauthors, the largest source of error was found to be inaccuracy of topographic corneal power measurements.[23]

The inaccuracy of topographic corneal power measurement could be related to the change of the anterior surface curvature and the reduction of corneal thickness. These corneal modifications alter the proportion between the radius of anterior and posterior surfaces of the cornea. In nonoperated eyes, the air-anterior surface interface (Dn = 1.376, r = 7.7 mm) produces a positive power of 48.8 D, and the posterior surface-aqueous humor interface (Dn = -0.04 = 1.336 - 1.376, r = 6.8 mm) produces a negative corneal power of –5.9 D.[24]

Computerized videokeratometers estimate the corneal power according to the anterior radius of curvature. The corneal power is determined by measuring the size of projected rings reflected off the anterior corneal surface. Image size is converted to radius of curvature or dioptric power using axial, instantaneous, and refractive formulas.[25,26,27] The standard refractive index used by these formulas is 1.3375. This theoretical value corresponds to the Gullstrand's model eye in which positive anterior corneal power, negative posterior corneal power, and different refractive indexes of the various corneal layers are represented in a single refractive surface. However, after PRK or LASIK, the radius of anterior corneal surface is increased and the distance of the anterior and posterior corneal surface is decreased. Thus, the traditional value of 1.3375 may become insufficient. Holladay and Mandell recommend changing the refractive index for corneal power calculation after PRK from 1.3375 to 1.376, which is the refractive index of the anterior stroma.[28,29] This recommendation is based on the fact that photoablation concerns only the anterior surface of the stroma and does not alter the other corneal structures. The modified refractive index provides a smaller discrepancy between the spherical equivalent of manifest refraction and computerized videokeratography.

Hugger and associates have found that a refractive index of 1.408 would optimize the correlation between change in manifest refraction and effective refractive power of the central 3 mm of the cornea.[30] According to these observations, computerized videokeratography

Table 13-1

Keratometry Readings*

Eye	Axial Length	Calc IOL	Placed IOL	Final SE
1	27.17	15.0	17.5	+0.12
2	24.98	20.0	22.0	+0.63
3	24.98	19.0	19.0	+0.25
4	25.05	13.5	15.5	-0.38
5	26.96	18.5	20.5	+0.50

Before, 1 week, and 6 months after CE/IOL on patients with pervious RK showing variability of induced flattening.

Table 13-2

Calculated and Placed IOL:
The Need for Increased IOL Power to Achieve Emmetropia Compared to Calculated IOL With Regular Keratometry

Eye	Pre K	1-Week Ks	Final Ks
1	39.4	37.3	39.0
2	39.3	36.5	37.2
3	41.7	41.5	41.9
4	44.9	44.5	45.0
5	37.3	35.1	37.1

Note: Approximately 2 D of additional power to achieve emmetropic results is needed.

does not provide an accurate estimation of the effective corneal power and induces erroneous IOL power calculations in patients who have undergone PRK. Further refinements of refractive index are needed to increase the accuracy of refractive formulas.

Addition of a Fixed Additional Power to IOL

Since the preceding methods are often unpredictable, one commonly used method is to simply add an additional power to the IOL calculated in the usual manner with standard keratometry. The theory is that the keratometry is underestimated in a relatively predictable amount in all cases, and the addition of 1.5 to 2 D of additional power will result in an IOL of approximately the correct power. In Table 13-1 we see that the addition of 2 D to the IOL calculated with standard keratometry results in approximately plano prescriptions in the final refraction several months after surgery. This method is no more predictable than others and the results may vary widely from case to case, but a review of personal results may indicate the usefulness of this approach, as demonstrated in Table 13-1. It is important to evaluate the results at least 6 months after surgery since these cases often have an induced hyperopia that resolves slowly over time (Table 13-2).

Intraoperative IOL Adjustment

An innovative approach to the problem of proper IOL selection in the corneal refractive patient has been suggested by Dr. Sunalp.[31] He performs the cataract surgery under topical anesthesia and has a vision chart taped to the ceiling for a rough visual acuity immediately after the lens is implanted and the eye is reformed. Additionally, an assistant performs retinoscopy without touching the eye and, if necessary, the IOL power is adjusted. The method is referenced in a nonreferred publication (*Ocular Surgery News*) and no long-term results are reported, but the idea seems promising particularly with the availability of portable autorefractors. This intraoperative approach may well provide the missing information to obtain repeatable results in the post-RK patient.

IOL Power Calculations

The IOL power can be calculated with different types of formulas. These formulas take into account the measurements of corneal power, axial length, and estimation of anterior chamber depth. They can be divided into empirical regression and theoretic optical formulas. Newer generation theoretical formulas such as Hoffer Q, Holladay theoretic, and the nonlinear empirical SRK/T have proven to be unaffected by variations in axial length and corneal power.[32] Empirical SRK I and II formulas are less predictable in long and short eyes. The superiority of newer generation formulas is due to their accuracy in predicting the pseudophakic anterior chamber depth.[33,34,35,36] As such, regression formulas, such as the SRK I and II, are not the most appropriate formulas to estimate the IOLP after corneal refractive surgery. Third-generation formulas, such as the Holladay, Hoffer Q, and SRK/T, provide much more accuracy. Finally, personalization of these formulas using a combination of them in conjunction with the axial length of the eye may increase the accuracy. According to Hoffer, this personalized system recommends the Hoffer Q formula for eyes shorter than 22 mm, the Holladay for eyes between 24.5 and 26 mm, the SRK/T for eyes greater than 26 mm, and an average of the three formulas for eyes between 22 and 24.5 mm.[19]

Practical Consequences

As refractive surgery is performed in increasing numbers each year, patients expect excellent visual acuity without corrective lenses. The ophthalmologist will have to manage these expectations when cataract extraction has to be performed two or three decades after the corneal refractive surgery.

None of the described methods of corneal power calculation reach the ideal accuracy. Standard keratometric readings have a tendency to overestimate corneal power and thus induce a hyperopic refractive error after cataract surgery. After RK, the hyperopic shift may reach 6 D, is particularly pronounced during the first week, and progressively decreases during a 6-month period. The hyperopic shift is due to the post-cataract removal corneal edema, as well as, in part, to an inaccurate keratometric reading. Standard keratometers measure a steeper area than the effective corneal center in keratotomized eyes, thus underestimating the IOLP calculation and inducing a hyperopic postoperative error. A subtraction of approximately 1 D to the average keratometry may limit the inaccuracy of the IOL power calculation. Alternatively, as we discussed, one may also choose to add 1.5 to 2 D to the IOL calculated with standard keratometry.

The clinical history method is difficult to use practically, as often patients who have undergone refractive surgery have their cataract removed two or three decades later with the same surgeon. In these cases, the preoperative keratometric reading and refraction are not available. An ID card, including the type of refractive surgery, the preoperative keratometric reading, preoperative refraction, and the postoperative refraction at some stable period should be systematically given to the patient. This information would certainly be beneficial for the patient and would allow us to compare this method to other ones.

The hard contact lens method is theoretically seducing; however, the IOL power calculation becomes inaccurate if the cataract is dense or responsible for a myopic shift.

Computerized videokeratography, in spite of its diagnostic interest to manage preoperative and postoperative refractive patients, has resulted in overestimation of corneal power. Further studies are needed to more precisely determine the correct value of the refractive index of the cornea that can be used in the calculation of IOL power after corneal refractive surgery. In addition, the refractive index after corneal refractive surgery may vary with the type of refractive procedure and on an individual basis.

After RK, computerized videotopography has shown to be superior to standard keratometric reading, as it estimates the effective corneal power by averaging more corneal points closer to the apex. These measurements have been obtained at the 3-mm zone of the topography.

After PRK or LASIK, the refractive index may vary in function of the curvature of the different surfaces of the cornea, the thickness of the ablated cornea, the composition of the epithelium, and Bowman's layer. These parameters may vary from patient to patient and their correlation with the accuracy of IOL power calculations needs to be clarified. The intraoperative adjustment of IOL power is time-consuming, and the connection between intraoperative vision and refraction has not been defined.

Postoperative Changes

After surgery, the patient with a previous RK may experience a hyperopic shift that will result in a prolonged postoperative visual improvement. Even best-corrected vision can be affected, and certainly uncorrected vision will be affected with 1 to 2 D of hyperopia and/or associated astigmatism. Why these changes occur is not completely clear, but some possibilities include elevated pressure during the procedure that stretches the incisions, corneal edema (although the effect may last for several months), and/or softening of the incisions with postoperative steroid administration. The effect certainly depends on incision healing. Patients with more than eight incisions, crossing incisions, inclusions in the incisions, significant diurnal variation, and/or any signs of corneal instability will have more problems than other patients without these signs and symptoms. Because topical steroids can affect the RK incisions and possibly extend the time to resolve the hyperopic shift, we limit their use to 1 week or less. One problem that can induce corneal instability is the intersection of the cataract incision with the previous RK or relaxing incisions (Figures 13-7a and b). In this patient, a previous relaxing incision was intersected with the corneal portion of the blue line incision. Since the relaxing incision was about 80% depth, this left little tissue holding the cornea in place and significant postoperative flattening occurred. Approximately 6 D of astigmatism resulted (flat axis in the direction of the incision), which resolved slowly over a period of 6 months. The same effect can be seen if a previous corneal transplant is present

Figure 13-7a. Topographic appearance 1 month after "C" procedure for 5 D of regular astigmatism and before clear lens exchange surgery.

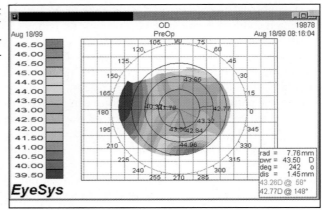

Figure 13-7b. Topographic appearance of the same patient 1 day after cataract surgery with intersection of the superior corneal relaxing incision and the corneal portion of a blue line incision showing induction of 6 D of irregular astigmatism.

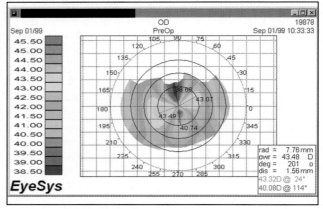

and the clear corneal or blue line incision intersects the graft margin. Care must be taken to end the anterior entrance of the cataract incision into the anterior chamber before it intersects with the graft margin. Intersection can cause immediate induction of a large amount of astigmatism, as in the case study, and in some cases will not resolve without through and through suturing or a wedge resection.

In Figures 13-8a through e, we show a case of cataract surgery after a previous RK with immediate 1-day induced hyperopia and subsequent resolution of that hyperopia over a 1-year period. This case was chosen to show the significant changes that can occur with lens-based surgery after RK. Observing the difference plots, we can see the approximately 3 D flattening with the original RK about 3 years before cataract surgery. Significant corneal flattening of about 4 D can be seen comparing preoperative to postoperative topographies and subsequent steepening of about 3.5 D to near the original corneal curvature over time. The graphs (see Figures 13-8d and e) show these changes in more detail over time. Tables 13-1 and 13-2 show different selected cases demonstrating the variability that can occur and the average errors seen with the use of "standard" keratometry. The calculated IOL powers were obtained using keratometry with an automated Humphery keratometer, showing that the "true" IOL power must usually be larger due to central corneal flattening, measured poorly with standard keratometry. The problem is that the error is variable depending on a variety of often undetermined factors. The tables also show the variability of the postoperative flattening, sometimes significant and sometimes virtually without hyperopic shift.

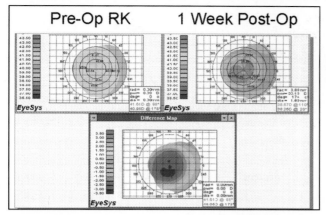

Figure 13-8a. Difference topographic plot between preoperative RK and 1-week postoperatively showing an approximate 3 D central flattening.

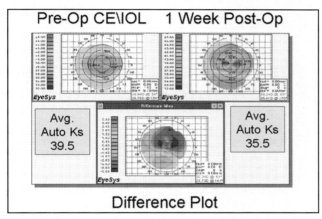

Figure 13-8b. Difference topographic plot of the same patient before and after cataract surgery showing induced flattening and induced astigmatism after the surgery.

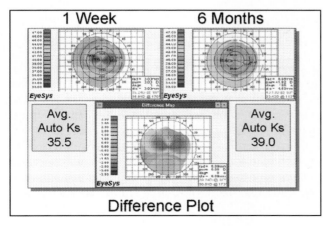

Figure 13-8c. Difference topographic plot between 1 week and 6 months showing resolution of induced flattening and induced astigmatism over time.

Figure 13-8d. Average keratometry over time showing immediate postoperative corneal flattening and its eventual resolution.

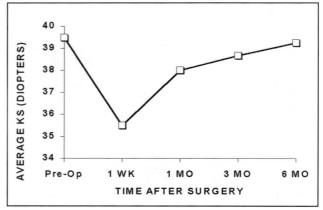

Figure 13-8e. Spherical equivalent over time with uncorrected vision showing immediate postoperative induced hyperopia and subsequent improvement of uncorrected vision over time.

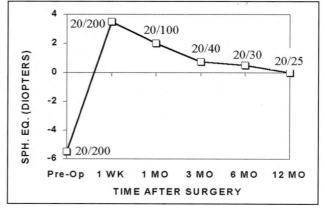

Summary

Clear lens exchange or cataract surgery after corneal refractive surgery can be a challenging procedure. It is important to consider not only overestimation of corneal power, but also the prospect of corneal instability. Proper preoperative patient counseling is essential to avoid patient discontent, and an understanding of the long-term nature of potential corneal power shifts is necessary to avoid premature intervention. In many cases of corneal instability, lens-based correction may avoid further corneal surgery and poor outcomes related to that intervention, but the corneal instability may continue. If the estimation of a continued hyperopic shift of approximately 1 D for every 10 years proves correct, additional refractive intervention may be necessary in the future no matter how accurate the cataract or lens exchange becomes.

References

1. Markovits AS. Extracapsular extraction with posterior chamber intraocular lens implantation in postradial keratotomy patient. *Arch Ophthalmol*. 1986;104:329.

2. Koch DD, Liu JF, Hyde LL, Rock RL, Emery JM. Refractive complications on cataract surgery after radial keratotomy. *Am J Ophthalmol*. 1989;108:676-682.

3. Siganos DS, Pallikaris IG, Lambropoulos JE, Koufala CJ. Keratometric readings after photorefractive keratectomy are unreliable for calculating IOL power. *J Refract Surg*. 1996;12:S278-279.

4. Holladay JT. Consultations in refractive surgery. *Refract Corneal Surg*. 1989;5:203.

5. Buzard KA. Consultations in refractive surgery. *Refract Corneal Surg*. 1989;5:202.

6. Soper JW, Goffman J. Contact lens fitting by retinoscopy. In: Soper JW, ed. *Contact Lens Advances in Design, Fitting, Application*. Miami, Fla: Symposia Specialist; 1974: 99.

7. Bogan SJ, Maloney RK, Drews CD, Waring GO III. Computer-assisted videokeratography of corneal topography after radial keratotomy. *Arch Ophthalmol*. 1991;109:834-41.

8. Buzard KA, Fundingsland BR. Treatment of irregular astigmatism with broad beam excimer laser. *J Refract Surg*. 1997;13:624-636.

9. Laranjeira E, Buzard KA. Pilocarpine in the management of overcorrection after radial keratotomy. *J Refract Surg*. 1996;12:382-90.

10. McDonnell PJ. Classification of corneal topography with videokeratography: corneal topography. In: Schanzlin DJ, Robin J, eds. *Measuring and Modifying the Cornea*. New York, NY: Springer-Verlag; 1992: 145-64.

11. Celikkol L, Pavlopoulos G, Weinstein B, Celikkol G, Feldman S. Calculation of intraocular lens power after radial keratotomy with computerized videokeratography. *Am J Ophthalmol*. 1995;120:739-750.

12. Quah BL, Wong KS, Tseng PS, Low CH, Tan DT. Analysis of photorefractive keratectomy patients who have not had PRK in their second eye. *Ophthalmol Surg Lasers*. 1996;27(5Suppl):S429-434.

13. Seitz B, Langenbucher A, Nguyen N, Kus M, Kuchle M. Underestimation of intraocular lens power for cataract surgery after myopic photorefractive keratectomy. *Ophthalmology*. 1999;106:693-702.

14. MacRae S, Rich L, Phillips D, Bedrossian R. Diurnal variation in vision after radial keratotomy. *Am J Ophthalmol*. 1989;107:262.

15. Waring GO, Lynn MJ, McDonnell PJ, PERK Study Group. Results of the prospective evaluation of radial keratotomy (PERK) study 10 years after surgery. *Arch Ophthalmol*. 1994;112:1298-1308.

16. Holladay JT. Cataract surgery in patients with previous keratorefractive surgery. *Ophthalmic Practice*. 1997;15:238-244.

17. Mandell RB. Corneal power correction factor for photorefractive keratectomy. *J Refract Corneal Surg*. 1994;10:125-8.

18. Holladay JT. IOL calculations following radial keratotomy surgery. *Refract Corneal Surg*. 1989;5:36A.

19. Hoffer KJ. Intraocular lens power calculation for eyes after refractive keratotomy. *J Refract Surg*. 1995;11:490-3.

20. Wilson SE, Klyce SD. Screening for corneal topographic abnormalities before refractive surgery. *Ophthalmology*. 1994;101:147-152.

21. Husain SE, Kohnen T, Maturi R, Hamadi E, Koch DD. Computerized videokeratography and keratometry in determining intraocular lens calculation. *J Cataract Refract Surg*. 1996;22:362-366.

22. Cuaycong MJ, Gay CA, Emery J, Haft EA, Koch DD. Comparison of the accuracy of computerized videokeratography and keratometry for use of intraocular lens calculation. *J Cataract Refract Surg.* 1993;19:S178-81.

23. Odenthal MTP, Van Marle GW, Pameyer JH. *Invest Ophthalmol Vis Sci.* 1996;37:S573.

24. Haigis W. Biometrie. In: Kampik A, et al. *Jahrbuch der Augenheilkunde.* Zulpicnk, Germany: Biermann; 1995; 123-40.

25. Klein SA, Mandell RB. Comparing shape and refraction powers in corneal topography. *Ophthalmol Vis Sci.* 1995;36:2096-2109.

26. Corbett MC, Marshall J, O'Bratt DPS, Rosen ES. New and future technology in corneal topography. *Eur J Implant Ref Surg.* 1995;7:267-273.

27. Mandell RB. The enigma of the corneal contour. CLAO J. 1992;18:267-273.

28. Holladay JT, Waring GO. Optics and topography of the cornea in RK. In: Waring GO, ed. *Refractive Keratotomy for Myopia and Astigmatism.* St Louis, Mo: Mosby-Year Book; 1992; 62.

29. Mandel RB. Corneal power correction factor for photorefractive keratectomy. *J Refract Corneal Surg.* 1994;10:125-128.

30. Hugger P, Kohnen T, La Rosa F, Holladay JT, Koch DD. Comparison of changes in manifest refraction and corneal power after photorefractive keratectomy. *Am J Ophthalmol.* 2000;129:68-75.

31. Sunalp MA. Use of intraoperative refractive refinement with piggyback IOL for difficult cataract cases. *Ocular Surgery News.* 1999;17(19):1-2.

32. Retzlaff JA, Sanders DR, Kraff MC. Development of the SRK/T intraocular lens implant power calculation formula. *J Cataract Refract Surg.* 1990;16:333-340.

33. Olsen T, Thim K, Corydon L. Accuracy of the newer generation intraocular lens power calculation formulas in long and short eyes. *J Cataract Refract Surg.* 1991;17:187-193.

34. Sanders DR, Rezlaff JA, Kraff MC. Comparison of the SRK/T formula and other theoretical and regression formulas. *J Cataract Refract Surg.* 1990;16:341-346.

35. Hoffer KJ. The Hoffer Q formula: a comparison of theoretical and regression formulas. *J Cataract Refract Surg.* 1990;16:341-346.

36. Holladay JT, Prager TC, Chandler TY. A three-part system for refining intraocular lens power calculations. *J Cataract Refract Surg.* 1990;16:341-346.

Index

BUILD *Your Library*

This book and many others on numerous different topics are available from SLACK Incorporated. For further information or a copy of our latest catalog, contact us at:

Professional Book Division
SLACK Incorporated
6900 Grove Road
Thorofare, NJ 08086 USA
Telephone: 1-856-848-1000
1-800-257-8290
Fax: 1-856-853-5991
E-mail: orders@slackinc.com
www.slackbooks.com

We accept most major credit cards and checks or money orders in US dollars drawn on a US bank. Most orders are shipped within 72 hours.

Contact us for information on recent releases, forthcoming titles, and bestsellers. If you have a comment about this title or see a need for a new book, direct your correspondence to the Editorial Director at the above address.

Thank you for your interest and we hope you found this work beneficial.